Critical Care of the Newborn

W. ALAN HODSON, M.D.

Professor and Head,
Division of Neonatal and
Respiratory Diseases,
Department of Pediatrics,
University of Washington

WILLIAM E. TRUOG, M.D.

Associate Professor,
Division of Neonatal and
Respiratory Diseases,
Department of Pediatrics,
University of Washington

W.B. SAUNDERS COMPANY

Philadelphia London Toronto
Mexico City Rio de Janeiro Sydney Tokyo

W. B. Saunders Company: West Washington Square
Philadelphia, PA 19105

1 St. Anne's Road
Eastbourne, East Sussex BN21 3UN, England

1 Goldthorne Avenue
Toronto, Ontario M8Z 5T9, Canada

Apartado 26370—Cedro 512
Mexico 4, D.F., Mexico

Rua Coronel Cabrita, 8
Sao Cristovao Caixa Postal 21176
Rio de Janeiro, Brazil

9 Waltham Street
Artarmon, N.S.W. 2064, Australia

Ichibancho, Central Bldg., 22-1 Ichibancho
Chiyoda-Ku, Tokyo 102, Japan

Library of Congress Cataloging in Publication Data

Hodson, W. Alan (William Alan), 1935–
Critical care of the newborn.

Includes index.
1. Neonatal intensive care. 2. Infants (Newborn)—Diseases. I. Truog, William E. II. Title. [DNLM: 1. Critical care—In infancy and childhood. 2. Infant, Newborn, Diseases—Therapy. WS 420 H692c]
RJ253.5.H63 1983 618.92'01 83-3369
ISBN 0-7216-1071-4

Critical Care of the Newborn ISBN 0-7216-1071-4

Last digit is the print number: 9 8 7 6 5 4 3 2

PREFACE

We wrote this book with the intention of providing a ready source of useful information for practicing physicians, hospital staff members, nurses, and students whose work brings them into contact with newborn infants who are critically ill or who have serious multisystem problems. We emphasize initial diagnostic approach and critical concepts of stabilization and management. We have tried not to duplicate information available in textbooks of neonatology and have focused on the more common and important illnesses. Pathophysiology and theoretical aspects of management are not emphasized.

Some of the approaches outlined herein may seem arbitrary. In fact, many are. This reflects the uncertainties that exist concerning optimal care for certain problems. Many of our recommendations are based on our own experience with patients in two affiliated special care nurseries that jointly admit approximately 1100 sick infants each year.

We hope this book fills the need for a practical, convenient source of information—for specialist and nonspecialist alike—for dealing with the sometimes overwhelming and complex medical problems of the newborn.

ACKNOWLEDGMENTS

The authors wish to thank Mary O'Leary, M.S., R.D., for her substantial and important contributions to Chapter 8, Nutrition and Fluid Administration.

We thank also our able administrative and secretarial staff, whose help in assembling this book was invaluable—Karen McMasters, B.J. Hayes, and JoAnn Jarrett, and extend most heartfelt thanks to Jan Livingston.

Finally, we thank our colleagues in the Division of Neonatal and Respiratory Diseases and others in the Department of Pediatrics of the University of Washington School of Medicine, who provide the superb and disciplined environment for the care of sick and vulnerable infants, who teach the principles of newborn medicine, and who provide a forum for clinical and basic research aimed at rendering much of this book obsolete.

W. ALAN HODSON
WILLIAM E. TRUOG

List of Abbreviations Frequently Used in This Book

AAP	American Academy of Pediatrics
ACD	acid citrate dextrose
ADH	antidiuretic hormone
AGA	appropriate for gestational age
Ao	aortic
ASD	atrial septal defect
ATP	adenosine triphosphate
A-V	arteriovenous
AVR	anomalous venous return
BAER	brain stem auditory evoked potential
BPD	bronchopulmonary dysplasia
BUN	blood urea nitrogen
BV	blood volume
C	centigrade
Ca	calcium
cal	calorie
cc	cubic centimeter
CHD	congenital heart disease
CHF	congestive heart failure
cm	centimeter
CMV	cytomegalovirus
CNS	central nervous system
CPD	citrate phosphate dextrose
CSF	cerebrospinal fluid
CT	computerized tomography
CVH	combined ventricular hypertrophy
CXR	chest x-ray
DES	diethylstilbestrol
DIC	disseminated intravascular coagulation
dL	deciliter
D10W	10% dextrose in water
ECF	extracellular fluid
ECG	electrocardiogram
EDC	expected date of confinement
EEG	electroencephalogram
EFA	essential fatty acid
EFE	endocardial fibroelastosis
ESR	erythrocyte sedimentation rate
ET	endotracheal
Ex Vol	volume of blood to be removed and replaced
FFA	free fatty acid

FIO_2	fractional inspired oxygen concentration
Fr	French
g	gram
G	glucose
GI	gastrointestinal
G6PD	glucose-6-phosphate-dehydrogenase
HFOV	high frequency oscillatory ventilation
Hg	mercury
HGH	human growth hormone
HLA	human leukocyte antigen
HMD	hyaline membrane disease
HPL	human placental lactogen
hr	hour
HSV	herpes simplex virus
HV	high volume
IDM	infant of a diabetic mother
I:E	inspiratory-expiratory
IgA	immunoglobulin A
IM	intramuscular
IU	international unit
IUGR	intrauterine growth retardation
IV	intravenous
IVH	intraventricular hemorrhage
IVP	intravenous pyelogram
kcal	kilocalorie
kg	kilogram
L	liter
LAH	left atrial hypertrophy
LATS	long-acting thyroid stimulator
LBW	low birth weight
LGA	large for gestational age
LP	lumbar puncture
L/S	lecithin/sphingomyelin
LSB	left sternal border
LV	low volume
LVH	left ventricular hypertrophy
MAP	mean airway pressure
MAS	meconium aspiration syndrome
mcg	microgram
MCT	medium chain triglyceride
mEq	milliequivalent
mg	milligram
min	minute
mL	milliliter
mm	millimeter
mm^3	cubic millimeter
mo	month
MV	mechanical ventilation
Na	sodium

NEC	necrotizing enterocolitis
NICU	Neonatal Intensive Care Unit
nm	nanometer
NTE	neutral thermal environment
O_2	oxygen
Obs. Hct	observed or measured hematocrit level
OFC	occipital frontal circumference
OR	operating room
OSM	osmol
oz	ounce
P_2	pulmonic second sound
PA	pulmonary artery
$PaCO_2$	partial arterial carbon dioxide pressure
PaO_2	partial arterial oxygen pressure
PBF	pulmonary blood flow
PC	Polycose
PDA	patent ductus arteriosus
PEEP	positive end-expiratory pressure
PFC	persistent fetal circulation
PIE	pulmonary interstitial emphysema
P-K	pyruvate kinase
PMN	pneumomediastinum
PPC	pneumopericardium
prn	as circumstances may require
PT	prothrombin time
$P_{tc}CO_2$	transcutaneous carbon dioxide pressure
$P_{tc}O_2$	transcutaneous oxygen pressure
PTT	partial thromboplastin time
PTU	propylthiouracil
PUFA	polyunsaturated fatty acid
PVR	pulmonary vascular resistance
q	every
qo	every other day
$Q\text{-}_0T_c$	corrected $Q\text{-}_0T$ interval
RBC	red blood count
RDA	recommended daily allowance
RSV	respiratory syncytial virus
RV	right ventricular
RVH	right ventricular hypertrophy
SAH	subarachnoid hemorrhage
sec	second
SEH	subependymal hemorrhage
SG	specific gravity
SGA	small for gestational age
SGOT	serum glutamic-oxaloacetic transaminase
SGPT	serum glutamic-pyruvic transaminase
SIADH	inappropriate antidiuretic hormone syndrome
SIDS	sudden infant death syndrome
T_3	triiodothyronine

T_4	thyroxine
TBG	thyroxine-binding globulin
TBPA	thyroxine-binding prealbumin
TBW	total body water
TE	tracheoesophageal
tid	three times a day
TORCH	toxoplasmosis, others, rubella, cytomegalovirus, herpes simplex virus
TPN	total parenteral nutrition
TSH	thyroid stimulating hormone
U	unit
UDP	uridine diphosphate
UDPG	uridine diphosphate glucose
VSD	ventricular septal defect
VUR	vesicoureteral reflux
WBC	white blood count

CONTENTS

INTRODUCTORY NOTE

The Saunders Blue Book Series is intended to provide, in a handy, convenient format, up-to-date information about therapy and patient care across a wide range of clinical fields. Blue Books are designed to help practicing physicians, nurses, emergency personnel, students, and other health care professionals deliver quality patient care.

Our series derives its title from the very first W.B. Saunders publication (Hare: *Essentials of Physiology*, Saunders, 1888). This book was part of a famous list of 24 *Question Compends* known as the "Blue Series." The purpose of that series was to sort out important scientific and clinical facts so that students could review and assess their knowledge. The name of the present series reflects its heritage from that pioneering venture.

Today, when scientific information is growing exponentially, health professionals recognize an increasing obligation both to remain current and to select from this sea of facts those that add significantly to the foundation upon which sound clinical practice is based. The Blue Books address this need. They should not be regarded as textbooks or office references, but as portable clinical tools—as vital to quality patient care as a stethoscope or blood pressure cuff.

MICKEY S. EISENBERG, M.D., PH.D.
Consulting Editor, Blue Book Series

1 FETAL MONITORING

GENERAL CONSIDERATIONS

Over the past 20 years, several new tests for assessing fetal well-being before and during labor have been developed. This chapter reviews the commonly used tests and the implications of their results in helping the physician to anticipate and to care for a depressed or asphyxiated newborn.

The principle behind screening for fetal well-being is that the severe fetal distress or placental insufficiency that produces fetal hypoxia is reflected in aberrations of the fetal heart rate and especially in episodes of bradycardia. Severe or persistent bradycardia not only signals fetal difficulty but also, because of the associated fall in fetal cardiac output, may lead to ever-worsening fetal acidosis and distress.

TESTS OF FETAL MATURITY PRIOR TO THE ONSET OF LABOR

Amniotic Fluid Analysis

In the management of a high-risk fetus it is often imperative to know the state of the patient's maturity and especially the maturity of the pulmonary system. The ratio of two phospholipids (lecithin and sphingomyelin) in a sample of amniotic fluid can be used to predict functional lung maturity and the absence of hyaline membrane disease, provided the L/S ratio is greater than 2.0 or 2.5:1, depending on the standards of each laboratory. These phospholipids are presumably produced by alveolar pneumocytes and secreted with fetal lung fluid up the airways and out the fetal mouth, whereupon they become part of the pool of amniotic fluid. A ratio lower than 2.5:1 is suggestive of lung immaturity and should alert the physician to the possibility of hyaline membrane disease developing in the newborn, if the infant is delivered within a few days of the analysis. The test is much more predictive of the absence of disease (if the ratio is normal) than the presence of disease (if the ratio is below normal).

Amniotic fluid can also be analyzed for creatinine concentration and for the presence of fetal epithelial cells that demonstrate a positive strain for fat content. Both tests give an indication of overall fetal maturity but are not predictive of specific pulmonary maturity.

TEST OF FETAL DISTRESS PRIOR TO THE ONSET OF LABOR

Nonstress Testing

A nonstress test involves abdominal wall indirect fetal heart rate monitoring for evidence of normal beat-to-beat variability, for the absence of severe decelerations in fetal heart rate (see next section for details), and for accelerations in fetal heart beat (greater than 15 beats per minute) occurring with fetal movement. This test is simple and rapidly performed, and it serves as a reasonably reliable screening exam for overall fetal well-being. When questions arise about the interpretation of this test, many centers utilize the oxytocin stress test.

Oxytocin Stress Test

An IV infusion of oxytocin is administered until 3 uterine contractions within 10 min have been induced. Again, external abdominal wall fetal heart rate monitoring is used to detect decelerations beginning more than 10 sec after the onset of a uterine contraction (late decelerations mean a positive test) or the absence of such decelerations in the presence of heart rate variability. The absence of decelerations indicates fetal well-being. A positive test suggests that the fetus is already compromised (there are many possible reasons) and has a poor chance of tolerating labor and vaginal delivery.

INTRAPARTUM TESTING FOR FETAL DISTRESS

Continuous Fetal Heart Rate Monitoring

Continuous electronic fetal heart rate monitoring coupled with continuous intra-amniotic cavity pressure monitoring may be used to detect the presence of abnormal fetal heart rate in association with the contractions, as in the oxytocin challenge test described above. The routine use of continuous electronic (versus intermittent auscultatory) monitoring for low-risk term pregnancies is controversial. The efficacy of continuous electronic monitoring in premature labor is currently being assessed in a randomized controlled study.

Several features of the fetal heart rate pattern are analyzed as labor progresses:

1. Intercontraction baseline heart rate (normal is 120–160 beats/min with premature infants more likely to be in the higher range of normal).
2. Degree of baseline minute-to-minute variability.

3. The presence or absence of acceleration in heart rate in response to fetal movement.
4. Deceleration of heart rate with contractions. Pay particular attention to the severity of the deceleration (slowing to less than 120 beats/min is moderate deceleration, slowing to less than 100 beats/min is severe deceleration).
5. Duration of the deceleration (longer than 30 sec to 1 minute is ominous).
6. The time of onset of the deceleration compared with the time of onset of the contraction. An early deceleration (beginning within 5 sec of the onset of the contraction) is considered to be a reflex due to head compression and is benign. Late deceleration, which begins more than 10 sec after the onset of the contraction or after the peak pressure of the contraction has been achieved, is an ominous sign and suggests uterine-placental insufficiency.
7. A variable deceleration (one of nonuniform shape, depth, and timing) may suggest cord compression but must be interpreted in light of the rest of the fetal heart rate tracing.
8. A sinusoidal heart rate pattern appears to correlate with severe fetal anemia and is therefore also an ominous pattern.
9. A "normal" fetal heart rate pattern is highly predictive of a normal transition to neonatal life for the fetus. An "abnormal" fetal heart rate pattern correlates rather poorly with neonatal outcome, perhaps because of the necessarily subjective nature of the interpretation.

Direct Fetal Scalp Capillary Blood Sampling for pH Assessment

This study can be performed with a vaginoscope using long capillary tubes, and it is indicated if an abnormal fetal heart rate pattern has been detected on monitoring. A fetal scalp pH of greater than 7.25 is considered normal during labor. Lower pH readings should be followed by repeat samplings at closely spaced (30- to 60-minute) intervals to determine the trend in pH for the fetus. Maternal hyperventilation or acidosis, respectively, will elevate or depress the fetal pH independently of any intrinsic fetal acidosis. Therefore, fetal pH monitoring must be interpreted in light of the presumed or measured maternal pH.

ADDITIONAL COMMENTS

The decision to terminate labor with a cesarean section or to persist with other treatments for an abnormal fetal heart rate pattern (maternal positioning, increased maternal fluids, maternal oxygen administration, or maternal sedation) must depend not only on the particular fetal heart rate pattern or scalp pH values but also on the trend over time toward a more worrisome pattern or a stable or improving pattern. Single isolated bits of information lifted from the sometimes confusing array of data available from these new techniques are insufficient in themselves to make such an important decision.

Other tests, such as urinary estriol measurement, are helpful only in following the well-being of the placental-fetal "unit" over the course of days or weeks and are therefore not discussed here. A newer maternal serum assay, human placental lactogen (HPL), produced in increasing amounts by the placenta as the pregnancy progresses, is easier to obtain and may be easier to interpret than the urinary estriols.

Newer techniques for discovering fetal distress, such as ultrasound assessment of fetal movement or transcutaneous fetal oxygen monitoring, may begin to play more of a role in prepartum or intrapartum monitoring in the future.

Visual interpretation of fetal heart rate patterns is prone to error, with either falsely normal or abnormal interpretations. This may partially account for the poor predictability of neonatal distress or asphyxia based on presumably ominous fetal heart rate patterns.

REFERENCES

1. Der Yuan D, Heinrichs WL, Ueland K: Fetal Management. In Kelley VC (ed): Practice of Pediatrics. New York, Harper and Row, 1981.
2. Epstein MF: Fetal Assessment. In Cloherty JP, Stark AR (eds): Manual of Neonatal Care. Boston, Little, Brown, 1980.
3. Hon EH, Koh S: Management of Labor and Delivery. In Avery GB (ed): Neonatology: Pathophysiology and Management of the Newborn. 2nd ed. Philadelphia, Lippincott, 1981.
4. James LS, Morishima HO, Daniel SS et al: Mechanism of late deceleration of the fetal heart rate. Am J Obstet Gynecol 113:578, 1972.

2 MATERNAL DRUG EFFECTS ON THE FETUS AND NEWBORN

DRUGS USED IN OBSTETRICS FOR MATERNAL ANALGESIA OR ANESTHESIA

Narcotics. Morphine, if administered intramuscularly, causes neonatal depression if the infant is delivered 2–4 hrs later. If injected intravenously, maximal depression of the neonate will occur if the infant is delivered 1 hr later. Infants will have absent or poor respiratory effort and depressed muscle tone. If narcotic-induced depression is suspected, administer naloxone (Narcan), 0.01 mg/kg IV.

Barbiturates. Administration of more than 8 mg/kg thiopental to the mother may produce depression (primarily respiratory) in the newborn.

Inhalation Anesthetics. These agents, such as halothane, may depress the infant if delivery occurs more than 20 min after administration of anesthesia. It will be necessary to provide assisted ventilation for the neonate as he also excretes the anesthetic agent via the lungs.

Local Anesthetics. The major risk to the fetus in using these substances is excessive concentration in fetal blood because of inappropriate dosage or site of injection. Seizures and respiratory depression may occur from the moment of birth. It is preferable not to deliver the infant immediately when maternal seizures are induced by these agents, as the fetus can eliminate the drug more rapidly into the maternal circulation across the placenta than by hepatic metabolism, which becomes the principal route of elimination after birth.

Magnesium Sulfate ($MgSO_4$). This agent may produce hypotonia and (rarely) respiratory depression in the newborn. Although blood levels may not correlate well with clinical findings, close observation is warranted if neonatal blood levels exceed 5 mEq/L.

Diazepam (Valium). This also can produce neonatal CNS depression if total maternal dosage exceeds 30 mg. Cases of typical neonatal withdrawal syndrome (see next section) have also been reported in infants following this degree of in utero exposure. Temperature instability may also occur in these infants.

The mainstay of therapy for the newborn is foreknowledge of the specific agents used in the mother *and* sufficient time to provide assisted ventilation to the newborn immediately upon delivery.

NEONATAL WITHDRAWAL SYNDROME

Mothers chronically addicted to narcotics or using methadone often deliver undergrown infants who may demonstrate signs of withdrawal during the first hours or days of life. These signs include jitteriness, sneezing, tremors, general irritability, extremely vigorous sucking movements, diarrhea, fever, and in about 3% of infants, seizures. Hyperventilation can produce respiratory alkalosis and a state of ionic hypocalcemia that may predispose to seizures. In addition, the problems characteristic of infants who are small for gestational age, such as hypoglycemia, can be expected.

The use of pharmacologic agents to treat the symptoms of drug withdrawal is based on subjective criteria. We use the findings of inability to feed and spontaneous awakening from sleep as signs to begin treatment. Treatment consists of phenobarbital in full antiseizure dosages. Duration of treatment must be individualized but may need to continue for weeks.

The same symptom complex may occur with chronic maternal use of ethchlorvynol (Placidyl), phencyclidine, barbiturates, glutethimide (Doriden), and ethanol. Methylphenidate (Ritalin), chlordiazepoxide (Librium), or methadone withdrawal by the infant may not begin until 2 weeks of age.

Other maternal agents producing immediate problems include the following. (This list must be viewed as incomplete as experience with new pharmaceutical agents produces new data.)

1. *Phenytoin and phenobarbital* may enhance the risk of vitamin K-dependent coagulation factor deficiency and cause generalized bleeding during the first day of life. Treatment of these infants should include extra parenteral vitamin K.
2. *Antithyroid medications* cross the placenta and may produce neonatal goiter and, rarely, respiratory distress secondary to airway obstruction. Goiter may also be induced by excessive maternal dosages of iodides (which are present in some antiasthmatic medications).
3. *Propranolol* may produce circulatory depression, bradycardia, hypotension, or hypoglycemia in the newborn.
4. *Isoxsuprine,* when given to suppress premature labor, may produce hypoglycemia if the infant is delivered within 2–4 hours of discontinuing the drug. There may also be increased risk of neonatal hypotension and tachycardia.

5. *Major tranquilizers* in mothers (e.g., chlorpromazine) have been associated with extrapyramidal neurologic signs in newborns, including facial grimacing, eye-rolling, and tremors. Lithium usage during pregnancy may result in hypothermia, cyanosis, bradycardia, and CNS depression in the newborn.
6. *Oral antidiabetic drugs* can produce neonatal hypoglycemia, and pregnant diabetic women generally are now treated with insulin to control their glucose levels.
7. *Oral antibiotics,* given for maternal urinary tract infections, may cross the placenta and produce hemolysis in infants with G6PD deficiency. Indirect hyperbilirubinemia and anemia will be the initial manifestations.

Some of these agents (e.g., alcohol, phenytoin) may produce teratogenic effects on the fetus in addition to the above immediate effects. Drug use by the mother during the first trimester should be avoided if at all possible, as this is the time of organogenesis and maximum fetal susceptibility to teratogens.

Multiple drug users, especially if methadone is one of the substances, appear to have an increased risk of thrombocytosis in their offspring, although the clinical importance of this effect is not at present clear. In addition, there appears to be an increased risk of sudden infant death syndrome in children of methadone users.

3

DELIVERY ROOM MANAGEMENT AND RESUSCITATION

GENERAL CONSIDERATIONS

The passage of an infant through the birth canal or a uterine incision can be a perilous beginning to extrauterine life. The physician responsible for the care of the newborn may need to intervene to reverse an asphyxiating process that begins minutes or hours prior to delivery. The reflex bradycardia that occurs as the fetus moves through the birth canal attests to the forces generated as the fetal head helps to dilate the cervix.

Resuscitation of a depressed newborn is most successful when there is adequate forewarning of trouble. This allows time to secure appropriate equipment and to consider any special procedures that may be necessary in the delivery room. Red blood cells may have to be obtained for immediate transfusion in cases of severe hemolytic disease, or suction equipment prepared for removal of aspirated meconium from the fetal airway.

There are few if any other situations in medicine where quick and efficient use of skills has a more profound impact on the life of the patient. Many developmental deficits and fixed motor disorders stem from perinatal problems.

The minimum necessary equipment for any delivery room is listed in Table 3–1.

Table 3–1. LIST OF EQUIPMENT NEEDED FOR RESUSCITATION

Table with overhead warmer and nonconductive mattress.
Source of oxygen.
Adequate lighting.
Infant stethoscope.
Adjustable suction apparatus with sterile catheters.
DeLee suction catheters.
Umbilical catheterization tray with 3½ and 5F polyvinyl chloride catheters.
Laryngoscope with infant-sized blades.
Cole tubes: 8, 10, and 12F.
Portex tubes: 2.5, 3.0, 3.5, and 4.0 mm internal diameter.
Rubber (anesthesia) bag with attachments for oxygen source.
Bennett and molded rubber face masks of several sizes.
Rubber bulb syringes.
Sterile syringes and needles, including butterfly needles.
Heparin for preparing syringes for blood gas determinations.
Black rubber oral airways: sizes 000, 00, and 0.
ECG monitor with easily placed leads.
Fresh bottles of glucose reagent sticks for heelstick glucose estimation.

PATHOPHYSIOLOGY

Decreased placental gas exchange, whether the result of decreased maternal uterine blood flow or umbilical cord compression, produces an elevation in fetal $PaCO_2$ and a decrease in PaO_2. Anaerobic metabolism ensues, with a metabolic acidosis superimposed on the respiratory acidosis. The result is asphyxia. The characteristic responses of the newborn to asphyxia and hypoxemia are apnea and bradycardia, with an ever-worsening imbalance and inadequacy of gas exchange and depression of pH.

Maternal and fetal problems associated with fetal distress are listed in Table 3–2.

Table 3–2. CONDITIONS CONTRIBUTING TO INCREASED RISK OF COMPLICATIONS OF LABOR OR DELIVERY

MATERNAL	FETAL
Young mother (<17)	Prematurity, breech, or transverse presentation
Older mother (>38), especially primiparous	Meconium staining of amniotic fluid
Diabetes mellitus	Twins in multiple gestation
Drug addiction	Large or small for gestational age
Toxemia of pregnancy	Evidence of fetal malformation from ultrasound or amniotic fluid examination
Placental abnormalities (abruption)	
Prolonged labor, first or second stage	
Adverse reproductive history	
Prolonged rupture of membranes	

OUTLINE OF AN INITIAL APPROACH TO THE DEPRESSED NEWBORN

Table 3–3. BIRTH: IMMEDIATE EVALUATION

Heart rate (count for 20 sec and multiply ×3)
Assess color
Assess respiratory effort
If heart rate is

≤50 beats/min	50–100 beats/min	≥100 beats/min
Absent respirations Color: cyanotic	Some respiratory efforts Color: cyanotic	
then	*then*	*then*
Immediate resuscitation. Dry the infant, suction the upper airway, apply bag-and-mask assisted ventilation. If there is no prompt response, then reclear the infant's airway and consider orotracheal intubation.	Dry the infant, suction airway, close observation with supplemental oxygen to face. If no improvement, bag-and-mask ventilation to begin by 1 min, or before if heart rate becomes progressively slower.	Dry the infant. If infant is cyanotic, use free-flowing oxygen to face. If no obvious respirations occur, stimulate the infant by rubbing his back or pinching the extremities for 20–30 sec. If heart rate starts to fall to less than 100 beats/min, institute bag-and-mask resuscitation.

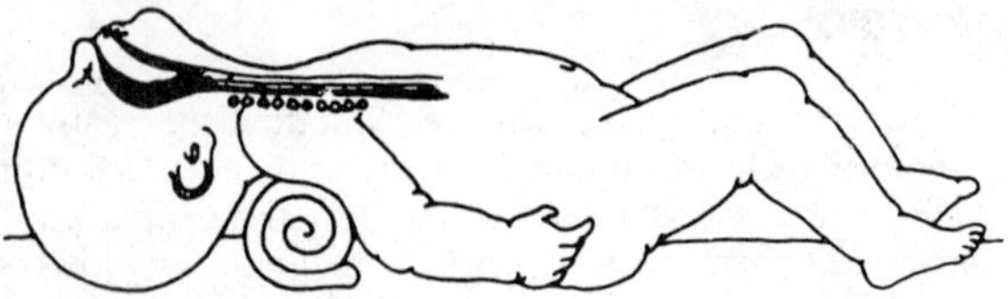

Figure 3–1. Proper positioning of an infant for ventilation by breathing bag and tightly fitting mask or for oral-tracheal intubation and bag and tube ventilation. The diaper roll is placed under the shoulders to allow adequate neck extension, overcoming the natural neck flexion that occurs upon supine positioning because of the baby's relatively large occiput.

Bag-and-mask ventilation as opposed to bag-and-tube ventilation is recommended as the initial step because it can be started more quickly, and gas exchange will occur with proper positioning of the infant's head (Fig. 3–1). The infant may respond following very few assisted breaths (<20), and all delivery room personnel can learn the procedure.

This flow scheme does not depend on obtaining a full Apgar score but rather focuses on the most critical and least subjective aspects of the infant's transition from fetal to neonatal life. For severely depressed infants, it is necessary to continue assisted ventilation and begin external massage (Fig. 3–2). This is done only when the heart rate remains below 60 beats/min after 1–2 min of *effective* ventilation. Then external compressions should commence at the rate of 120/min with the compressions delivered to the mid-sternum, depressing the sternum 1–2 cm with each compression (Fig. 3–2). The resuscitator's hands encircle the ba-

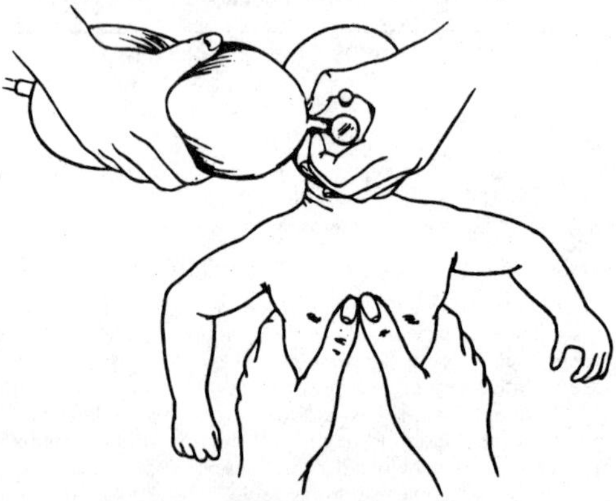

Figure 3–2. Cardiopulmonary resuscitation with bag and mask technique for ventilation and external cardiac massage with the thumbs of the second resuscitator applied at the midsternum.

Table 3–4. GUIDELINES FOR SELECTION OF ORAL AIRWAY, ENDOTRACHEAL TUBE, AND SUCTION CATHETER

WEIGHT (g)	ORAL AIRWAY	SIZE OF ENDOTRACHEAL TUBE (mm)	SIZE OF SUCTION CATHETER
<1000	000	2.5	5F
1000–1500	000	2.5 or 3.0	5 or 6F
1501–2500	00	3.0	6F
2501–3000	0	3.0 or 3.5	6 or 8F
>3000	0	3.5	8F

by's chest to help stabilize him, and the thumbs compress the sternum.

At this point, endotracheal (ET) intubation will often be a more effective means of delivering assisted ventilation. See Table 3–4 for a guide to ET tube size.

Infusion of Bicarbonate. (See Chapter 20.) An umbilical vein catheter is easiest to place in an emergency situation. An umbilical arterial catheter takes more time and can be placed, if needed, after the initial period of stabilization. The venous catheter can be used for infusion of bicarbonate if it is inserted just to the point of obtaining blood return. We recommend a single dose of 2–3 mEq/kg of bicarbonate infused at 1 mEq/min while resuscitation proceeds if ventilation and cardiac massage are needed for more than 1–2 min. Venous blood pH and $PaCO_2$ can also be obtained through a venous catheter and used as a rough guide for further therapy. Similarly, it is possible to place a No. 23-gauge butterfly needle into the umbilical vein and infuse drugs without actually cutting across the umbilical cord. These procedures require a second person to continue assisted ventilation.

Very rarely an infant will not respond to assisted ventilation, external massage, and bicarbonate even after 3–5 min of treatment. When this situation occurs, a single dose of epinephrine (0.1 mL/kg 1:10,000 dilution) should be administered either intravenously or through the endotracheal tube. Severe bradycardia is unlikely to be vagal in origin, and routine use of atropine injection in the delivery room is not recommended.

Other Comments

1. Do not administer bicarbonate without continuing assisted ventilation.
2. Establishing a patent airway is *the* critical step in effective resuscitation.
3. Ventilation with air or, better yet, 100% oxygen helps overcome elevated pulmonary vascular resistance (PVR) and results in an increased pulmonary blood flow.

Table 3–5. DRUGS USED IN RESUSCITATION OF THE NEWBORN

DRUG	INDICATION	DOSAGE
Sodium bicarbonate	Metabolic acidosis	2 mEq/kg initially
Dextrose	Low glucose	2 mL/kg 25% dextrose initially
Epinephrine hydrochloride	Bradycardia	0.1 mL/kg of 1:10,000 solution
Plasma-like substance (5% albumin in normal saline)	Low intravascular volume because of fetal-neonatal bleeding	15 mL/kg 5% solution
Naloxone (Narcan)	Respiratory depression secondary to maternal narcotic administration	0.01 mg/kg IV preferably or IM

4. Do not place the umbilical clamp so close to the skin of the umbilicus that it is impossible to insert a needle in the umbilical vein to inject drugs.
5. Table 3–5 provides a summary list of drugs useful in delivery room resuscitation.

ONGOING RESUSCITATION

1. Continued assisted ventilation.
2. IV line for glucose administration, especially in small or premature infants, as symptomatic hypoglycemia can occur rapidly (30–60 min) following asphyxia.
3. Provide a radiant heat source. Hypothermia occurs quickly during resuscitation.
4. Chest radiograph to determine if a pneumothorax has developed with assisted ventilation.

SPECIAL SITUATIONS

Meconium Aspiration. Aspirate meconium from pharynx (see Chapter 9).

Hypovolemic Shock. This may occur with maternal-placental or fetal bleeding. The infant will appear to be weak, floppy, and pale with barely palpable peripheral pulses. The immediate treatment is appropriate blood volume replacement (see Table 3–5 and Chapter 16) with close monitoring of vital signs and hematocrit reading. Expected normal blood pressure at birth is listed in Table 3–6.

Hydrops Fetalis. These infants often respond very slowly to resuscitative procedures and may have excessive pleural or peritoneal fluid that inhibits normal respiration.

Table 3–6. EXPECTED NORMAL BLOOD PRESSURE AT BIRTH*

	28–30 WEEKS	30–32 WEEKS	34–36 WEEKS	TERM
Systolic (torr)	48–52	52–55	60–62	62–65
Mean (torr)	32–35	38–40	42–46	45–50

*Pressure will gradually increase over first hours and days of life. Infants with hyaline membrane disease often have lower mean and peak pressures.

SIGNIFICANT BIRTH INJURIES

These usually occur in full term or large for gestational age infants.

Peripheral Nervous System

These injuries occur because of lateral flexion and traction of the neck to allow shoulder delivery.

1. *Brachial plexus injury.* Injury to 5th and 6th cervical spinal nerves (Duchenne-Erb paralysis). Affected arm is adducted; forearm is pronated; wrist is flexed; reflexes are absent locally; grasp reflex is intact. Treatment consists of prevention of further injury by immobilization, then passive range of motion exercises may be attempted after several days.
2. *Injury to 7th and 8th cervical and first thoracic spinal nerve (Klumpke's paralysis*). Muscles of hand are affected and grasp is absent.
3. *In some cases the entire brachial plexus is injured.* Management of 2. and 3. is similar to 1. Recovery is not always complete. Children in whom little or no recovery can be detected by 2 weeks have a much more guarded prognosis for complete recovery.
4. *Phrenic nerve injury* is usually associated with Duchenne-Erb paralysis. Diaphragmatic paresis or paralysis presents with tachypnea and occasionally results in respiratory failure, necessitating mechanical ventilation. Diagnosis can be confirmed by fluoroscopy. A major hazard is development of aspiration pneumonia. Plication of the diaphragm may be necessary if signs of recovery are not apparent by 1–2 weeks after birth.
5. *Facial nerve paresis* is usually caused by misapplication of forceps. The infant has an asymmetrical face while crying. This injury may produce an unblinking eyelid. The eye will then need protection with methyl cellulose eyedrops until lid function returns.

Central Nervous System

(See also Chapter 15.)

1. *Subdural hematoma* usually but not always occurs in the full term infant. There may be marked discrepancy between the clinical appearance of the infant and the degree of hemorrhage. Treatment of symptoms of localized pressure on the brain, if indicated, is by subdural aspiration of the blood. This may be done via the open fontanel and repeated frequently.
2. *Subarachnoid hemorrhage* can occur with difficult delivery and may cause seizures in children who otherwise appear well. Computerized tomography (CT) scanning will demonstrate the lesion.
3. The common finding of *cephalohematoma* is associated with a 5% incidence of underlying linear skull fracture. No radiograph or special treatment is necessary unless palpation suggests a depressed skull fracture. If this is found, a repeat radiograph several months later should be obtained to ascertain complete healing. Occasionally leptomeningeal cysts develop following incomplete resolution of the fracture.

Other Injuries

Bruising commonly occurs and may contribute to neonatal jaundice. Clavicular fractures are the most common musculoskeletal injury. Other fractures are rare.

REFERENCES

1. Anon: Advanced cardiac life support for neonates. JAMA 244:495, 1980.
2. Truog WE: Care of the Newborn in the Delivery Room. *In* Kelley VC (ed): Practice of Pediatrics. Hagerstown, Md., Harper and Row, 1979, vol. 1, ch. 83.
3. Vyas H, Milner A, Hopkins I, Boon A: Physiologic responses to prolonged and slow rise inflation in the resuscitation of the asphyxiated newborn infant. J Pediatr 99:635, 1981.

4

ASPHYXIA

GENERAL CONSIDERATIONS

Brain damage secondary to asphyxia is a major cause of morbidity and mortality during the neonatal period and a major contributor to long term serious sequelae such as mental retardation, seizures, and motor abnormalities, including cerebral palsy. It is the most common cause of major neurologic dysfunction in infants and older children. The terms asphyxia, hypoxia, and ischemia are more or less interchangeable since hypoxia and ischemia almost always occur together.

Etiology. Hypoxia can occur in utero, at the time of delivery, or postnatally as a consequence of cardiovascular or pulmonary disease. The most common problem is that associated with asphyxia during the intrapartum or delivery process. Respiratory causes include hyaline membrane disease, meconium aspiration, apnea, or hypoventilation due to obstructive airway disease associated with seizures or aspiration. Hypoxemia may occur as a consequence of severe right-to-left shunting due to persistent fetal circulation, cyanotic congenital heart disease, sepsis, hypotension, or shock with poor cerebral perfusion secondary to blood loss.

Pathogenesis. Decreased oxygen uptake through the placenta or the lungs or decreased oxygen delivery via the circulation results in damage to the brain tissues. Some areas may be more vulnerable than others due to the differences in autoregulation of the cerebral microcirculation. In general, it is believed that the vital areas of the brain (e.g., the brain stem) have much less of a decrease in blood flow than the cortical areas and therefore a less severe oxygen deficiency. Cerebral edema is a common consequence, occurring several hours after the asphyxial insult and probably secondary to altered capillary endothelial integrity and altered neuronal cell membrane permeability. The rate of glycolysis is transiently increased, as is lactate production. There is decreased production of adenosine triphosphate (ATP) and phosphocreatine.

Although the central nervous system effects of asphyxia are the most severe, other organ systems may also suffer. Cardiac impairment may be reflected in poor perfusion and blood pressure abnormalities (both hypotension and hypertension); pulmonary edema may develop and be reflected in hypoxemia and hypercarbia, possibly further impairing cerebral perfusion regulation; and renal dysfunction will be reflected in oliguria or anuria.

PRESENTATION

Intrauterine asphyxia may be associated with fetal heart rate abnormalities, presence of meconium, decreased fetal movement, scalp pH below 7.25, low Apgar score, prolonged rupture of membranes, prolonged labor, and difficult delivery. Postnatal asphyxia may be associated with single or multiple episodes of abnormal cardiorespiratory function such as apnea, severe pulmonary disease, severe congenital heart disease, or obstructive airway disease.

First 12 Hours of Life

During the first hours of life, the infant appears flaccid and stuporous, with little movement or tone, and may be comatose. Breathing is often irregular and characterized as episodic or periodic. The eyes move in a disconjugate fashion. Pupils usually react to light. Abnormal movements such as eye blinking, horizontal eye movements, lip smacking, sucking movements, bicycling movements of the legs, or flailing of the arms can be subtle signs of seizures. Half of all seizures due to asphyxia are characterized by tonic movements. Generalized or multifocal seizures will occur in 50% of all infants before the first 12 hours of life. Seizure activity may be delayed up to 36 hours. The signs of central nervous system hypoxia vary with the gestational age of the newborn infant, and are, of course, much more subtle in the low birth weight or premature infant.

Second 12 Hours of Life

This period is characterized by increased alertness, with the eyes appearing constantly open or "staring." The baby has a worried expression and appears anxious and perhaps jittery. Increasing irregularity of breathing may occur with frank apneic episodes. The muscle tone is usually diminished over that of the first 12 hours.

1 to 3 Days of Age

Depending on the severity of the asphyxia, there may be a decreasing level of consciousness with loss of some cranial function, including abnormal eye movements, loss of pupillary reaction to light, and absent "doll's eye" reflex. More profound central nervous system depression may be associated with an intraventricular hemorrhage in a premature baby or a subarachnoid hemorrhage in a full term infant. The fontanel may become increasingly tense with a sudden change in neuromotor activity.

After 3 Days

Often after 3 days, the infant begins to show gradual improvement with evidence of subsiding cerebral edema. Full term infants will be slow to begin feeding and will have a weak suck and increased pharyngeal secretions, which tend to obstruct the airway. There will be a weak, high-pitched cry. The infant will remain somewhat flaccid, with a decreased Moro response. The deep tendon reflexes may be normal. The tongue will often show vesiculation, and the mandible will fall posteriorly.

DIAGNOSIS

History

The historical information is the most critical in determining the cause and severity of an asphyxial episode. Pertinent information includes all factors affecting the in utero environment, labor and delivery, immediate adaptation to birth measured by the Apgar score, and subsequent postnatal adaptation.

Laboratory Evaluation

EEG. Usually nonspecific with much variability, but it is important to establish a baseline pattern. Serial studies commonly reveal a progression: decreased voltage and frequency → periodic bursts of sharp and slow waves → periodic pattern ("burst-suppression" pattern) → further voltage suppression → isoelectric.

Cranial Ultrasound. Especially important in premature infants to detect intraventricular hemorrhage.

Computerized Axial Tomography. To rule out subarachnoid hemorrhage.

Technetium-99 Scan. Areas of increased uptake indicate extent of brain injury. The scan also determines basal ganglia injury, and may provide prognostic information. Optimum time = 1 week.

Lumbar Puncture. Increased red blood cells, increased white blood cells, increased protein, and increased pressure are often found. Lactate level in CSF may be helpful.

Intracranial Pressure. Tense and bulging fontanel. Continuous monitoring with an anterior fontanel sensor would be useful but is not yet reliable.

Serum Electrolytes. Inappropriate antidiuretic hormone syndrome (SIADH) may occur following asphyxia. Serum sodium is decreased; serum osmolarity is decreased; urine osmolarity is increased.

Brainstem Auditory Evoked Potential (BAER). Often shows absence of 5th wave. More than 50% of asphyxiated infants will have an abnormal BAER, most often returning to normal. There is insufficient information regarding prognosis to warrant general use.

TREATMENT

Supportive Care

Respiratory

1. Oxygen to prevent further hypoxia during a seizure or secondary to prolonged apnea. Continuous supplemental oxygen may be necessary. Assess by transcutaneous oxygen monitoring.
2. In severely obtunded infants, mechanical ventilation may be necessary to maintain oxygenation. Mechanical ventilator settings to produce hyperventilation with a $PaCO_2$ of 30 ± 3 mm Hg may have a beneficial effect on brain edema by diminishing cerebral blood flow.

Cardiovascular

Since asphyxia may impair autoregulation of cerebral blood flow, it is important to monitor blood pressure as a rough guide to cerebral perfusion. Attempt to maintain mean blood pressure above 40 mm Hg in full term infants and over 30 mm Hg in preterm infants. Because of the possibility of endocardial damage, contractility may be transiently depressed and vasopressors may be required to maintain blood pressure. However, the effects of asphyxia on blood pressure are not easily predicted, and rapid fluctuations may occur in the patient.

Intravenous Glucose and Water

There is considerable controversy about the brain metabolism of glucose following asphyxia and the appropriate fluid administration to maintain cerebral perfusion yet minimize cerebral edema. Lactate-pyruvate levels remain high after asphyxia, so IV glucose may increase brain lactate levels; however, a substrate will be needed. $D_{10}W$ at 70 mL/kg/day is recommended, with individualization of electrolyte supplementation.

Intravenous fluid requirements will also depend on the presence of asphyxia-induced renal failure and oliguria. This usually resolves 3–4 days after birth.

Phenobarbital

Preventive

There is much controversy regarding the use of high doses of phenobarbital (e.g., 20 mg/kg IM or 10 mg/kg IV × 2) prior to the onset of seizures to reduce cerebral metabolism, reduce localized cerebral vasoconstriction, prevent or reduce edema, and remove free oxygen radicals. Use depends on clinical circumstances and severity of asphyxia.

Seizures

Give 20 mg/kg/IV in 2 doses of 10 mg/kg over 5–10 minutes. Maintenance: 5–10 mg/kg/day, decreasing over 4 days to 3–4 mg/kg/day depending on control of seizures and neurologic status and frequent checks of serum level. Therapeutic level is 20–30 mcg/mL.

Other Anticonvulsants

Add phenytoin if phenobarbital is unsuccessful after 4–6 hours. See Chapter 15 for treatment of seizures.

Glucocorticoids

No proven value. Not recommended.

Mannitol

No proven value. May increase risk of intracranial hemorrhage in premature infants.

ADDITIONAL COMMENTS

1. Asphyxia presents a wide spectrum of clinical disorders, depending on severity and gestational age.
2. Many aspects of treatment remain controversial; however, they should focus on preventing further damage.
3. Prognosis will depend on severity of insult. If seizure episodes are multiple or prolonged, the outlook is poor. If the infant remains neurologically abnormal at the time of discharge, the outlook is poor. A normal neurologic examination at 1 year does not rule out subsequent neuro-intellectual abnormalities.

REFERENCES

1. Brann HW, Dykes FD: Effects of intrauterine asphyxia on the full term neonate. Clinics in Perinatology 4(1):149, 1977.

2. Cassady G: Pathophysiologic Picture of the Postasphyxiated Infant. *In* Peckham GJ, Hegmann MA (eds): Cardiovascular Sequelae of Asphyxia in the Newborn. 83rd Ross Conference on Pediatric Research. Columbus, Ohio, Ross Laboratories, 1982, p. 66.
3. Hill A, Volpe JJ: Hypoxic-ischemic brain injury in the newborn. Seminars in Perinatology 6:25, 1982.
4. Lees MH: Perinatal asphyxia and the myocardium. J Pediatr 96:675, 1980.

5

ASSESSMENT OF GESTATIONAL AGE

GENERAL CONSIDERATIONS

In the overall assessment of newborn infants it is important to determine gestational age and the appropriate intrauterine growth for that age, whether the infant is premature (<37 completed weeks of gestation), term (38–42 weeks), or postmature (>42 weeks). It is particularly important to detect small for gestational age (SGA) infants, since they will have a different set of problems than those infants with low birth weight because of prematurity alone.

PRESENTATION

History

1. Last menstrual period and expected date of confinement (EDC).
2. Time fetal heart tones first heard (18–22 weeks).
3. Fetal quickening (16–18 weeks).
4. Fundal height.
5. Fetal ultrasound: biparietal diameter. If SGA is suspected, ratio of circumference of head to abdomen is important to determine.

Clinical

1. Birth weight, length, occipital-frontal circumference (OFC).
2. Neurologic criteria (see chart).
3. External physical criteria (see chart).

The scoring system provides accuracy to within 2 weeks after 30 weeks of gestation and less accurate correlation prior to 28 weeks. The method is also reliable between 6 and 60 hours after birth. The criteria used in the following chart are taken from Ballard, Novak, and Driver (1979).

Notes on Exam for Neuromuscular Activity

Posture. Assess when the infant is quiet and supine.

Square Window. Flex the baby's hand between the thumb and index finger. Measure the angle between the hypothenar eminence and the forearm.

Arm Recoil. Hold the forearms flexed for 5 seconds; then extend forearms; then release. Assess degree of recoil toward flexed position.

Neuromuscular Maturity

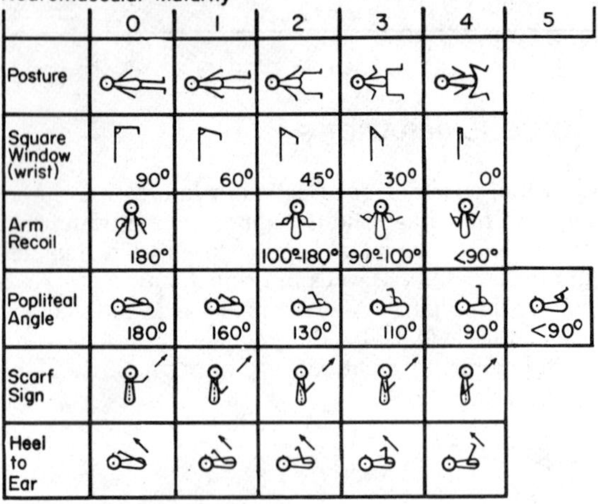

Physical Maturity

	0	1	2	3	4	5
Skin	gelatinous red, trans-parent	smooth pink, vis-ible veins	superficial peeling, &/or rash few veins	cracking pale area rare veins	parchment deep cracking no vessels	leathery cracked wrinkled
Lanugo	none	abundant	thinning	bald areas	mostly bald	
Plantar Creases	no crease	faint red marks	anterior transverse crease only	creases ant. 2/3	creases cover entire sole.	
Breast	barely percept.	flat areola no bud	stippled areola 1-2mm bud	raised areola 3-4mm bud	full areola 5-10mm bud	
Ear	pinna flat, stays folded	sl. curved pinna; soft c̄ slow recoil	well-curv. pinna; soft but ready recoil	formed & firm c̄ instant recoil	thick cartilage ear stiff	
Genitals ♂	scrotom empty no rugae		testes descend-ing few rugae	testes down good rugae	testes pendulous deep rugae	
Genitals ♀	prominent clitoris & labia minora		majora & minora equally prominent	majora large minora small	clitoris & minora completely covered	

Figure 5–1. A scoring scale for neuromuscular maturity and physical maturity. See notes in the text for details of assessing neuromuscular maturity. After adding the points scored, the estimated gestational age can be determined using Table 5–1, the maturity rating table.

Popliteal Angle. With baby's pelvis flat, hold the thigh in the knee-chest position. Then extend lower leg from the knee until resistance is met. Measure the angle.

Scarf Sign. With baby supine, take one hand and try to place it posteriorly around the neck of the contralateral shoulder. Lift the elbow across the body. See how far the elbow will go across the body.

Heel to Ear. With baby supine, move the baby's foot toward the ipsilateral ear. Observe remaining distance to ear and extension of knee.

To estimate gestational age, add the total points from the chart and compare the total to the corresponding score on the maturity rating table (see Table 5–1). Determination of SGA, large for gestational age (LGA), or appropriate for gestational age (AGA) growth status can then be made by reference to appropriate infant weight grids, available in any nursery.

For more detail, see Dubowitz and Dubowitz (1977).

Table 5–1. MATURITY RATING

SCORE	WEEKS
5	26
10	28
15	30
20	32
25	34
30	36
35	38
40	40
45	42
50	44

SMALL FOR GESTATIONAL AGE INFANTS

There are many causes for intrauterine growth failure, defined as a birth weight beneath two standard deviations of expected normal for gestational age. Determination of gestational age provides clues that may be important in treatment, diagnosis, and prognosis, particularly in the low birth weight group. SGA infants have a greater number of cells per unit mass, and hence their metabolic expenditures and caloric needs are greater.

In utero infections, nutritional inadequacies, and poor placental oxygenation all have important long-range implications. There is also a high incidence of congenital malformations in SGA infants. Hypoglycemia with decreased glycogen stores is a particularly common problem.

ETIOLOGY

Maternal Factors

1. Chronic hypertension.
2. Chronic renal disease.
3. Cigarette smoking.
4. Severe diabetes.
5. Toxemia.
6. Maternal hypoxia (altitude, hemoglobinopathies, chronic lung disease).
7. Poor nutrition.
8. Drug abuse, alcohol.

Placental and Uterine Factors

1. Vascular anomalies (hemangioma, abnormal cord insertion).
2. Bicornuate uterus.
3. Infarction of placenta.
4. Twin-twin transfusion (donor twin usually smaller).
5. Partial placental separation.

Fetal Factors

1. Twins.
2. Chromosomal abnormalities.
3. Congenital malformations.
4. Infections (rubella, cytomegalovirus, toxoplasmosis, syphilis, herpes).

MANAGEMENT

1. Prenatal assessment of fetal well-being and rate of growth, including ultrasonic search for congenital defects.
2. Search for and treat associated congenital defects.
3. Screen for and treat hypoglycemia through 72 hours of age.
4. Determine hematocrit and treat hyperviscosity (see Chapter 16).
5. Environmental temperature needs may be less than those of normally grown infants of comparable weight owing to metabolic mass.
6. Caloric requirements may be greater than those of normally grown infants of comparable gestational age.
7. Fluid requirements/kg may be less than those of a normally grown infant of the same weight.

ADDITIONAL COMMENTS

1. Among SGA infants there is a moderately high risk of impaired postnatal growth and development, depending on the cause and duration of intrauterine growth retardation. Infants with long-

standing intrauterine growth retardation (through the last ⅔ of pregnancy) associated with reduced head growth are at high risk for developmental disabilities.

2. Velocity of growth after birth is a more important prognosticator of subsequent growth potential than intrauterine growth.
3. The high incidence of perinatal asphyxia probably contributes to increased developmental difficulties.
4. The cause rather than the fact of growth retardation at birth is of greatest significance in long term outcome.

REFERENCES

1. Ballard J, Novak K, Driver M: A simplified score for assessment of fetal maturation of newly born infants. J Pediatr 95:769, 1979.
2. Dubowitz LMS, Dubowitz V: Gestational Age of the Newborn—A Clinical Manual. Reading, Mass., Addison-Wesley, 1977.
3. Narayanan I, Dua K, Guiral VV, Mehta DK, Mathew M, Prabhakar AK: A simple method of assessment of gestational age in newborn infants. Pediatrics 69:27, 1982.

6

RECOGNITION OF CONGENITAL MALFORMATIONS

GENERAL CONSIDERATIONS

A detailed review and catalog of the common congenital malformations is beyond the scope of this book. Such information is readily available in the references listed at the end of this chapter. Rather, an outline of a systematic approach to diagnosis will be presented here.

Congenital malformations recognizable at birth are relatively common, occurring in at least 1 in 400 liveborn infants.

Not all serious defects can be diagnosed at birth. Examples of commonly undetected defects include ventricular septal defects and some chromosomally determined anomalies, such as XYY, XXY (Klinefelter's syndrome), and XO (Turner's syndrome).

It is important to bring the unsettling news of the discovery of a congenital malformation to the parents' attention as quickly as possible. Any delay will undermine their ultimate confidence in the physicians at a difficult time.

APPROACH TO THE CHILD WITH A MALFORMATION

History

1. Prior children with malformations or with a history of abortions, stillbirths, or neonatal deaths in the family.
2. Maternal drug exposure during pregnancy, including nonprescription drugs, aspirin, old antibiotics she may have taken and forgotten, iodine-containing compounds, perhaps even the mother's own in utero drug exposure, as, for example, to diethylstilbestrol (DES).
3. Signs of abnormal fetal development—no fetal movement, frequent bleeding.
4. Parental age—older maternal age (>35) increases risk of Down's syndrome; older paternal age is associated with several autosomal dominant lesions.

PHYSICAL EXAMINATION

1. In addition to obvious anomalies (e.g., omphalocele, cyanotic heart disease), it is important to note other features to define the full extent of the lesions.
2. Note gestational age at birth. Children with tracheo-esophageal fistula are very commonly born prematurely and may have other complex malformations.
3. SGA status: many have chromosome defects, e.g., Down's syndrome or other trisomies. LGA status: infants of diabetic mothers (IDM) have an increased incidence of congenital malformations (5–10%).
4. Examination of the head and face, noting several features:
   a. Low-set hair line; aberrantly located hair whorl.
   b. Hypo- or hypertelorism; corneal opacities.
   c. Mid-face and nasal development.
   d. Development of philtrum and lips.
   e. Location and size of the external ear; degree of infolding of helix.
   f. Presence of cleft lip and/or cleft palate.
   g. Coloboma of iris.
   h. Mandibular development.
   i. Presence of sinuses or skin tags, especially in preauricular region.
   j. Evidence of closed cranial sutures.
   k. Overall shape and characteristic features of face ("triangular," "coarse").
   l. Abnormal angulation of palpebral fissure.
5. Extremities—note for:
   a. Extra or missing digits.
   b. Digital overlapping.
   c. Digitalization of the thumbs (thumbs have the appearance of the other fingers on the hand).
   d. Length and symmetry of extremities.
   e. Development of nail beds.
   f. Tightness or fixed position of joints.
   g. Dermal ridge patterning; palmar crease pattern.
6. Genitalia—overall development, degree of masculinization or feminization, and evidence of aberrant urethral opening.
7. Other physical features:
   a. Anal position on perineum.
   b. Number of umbilical arteries.
   c. Presence of abnormal hypo- or hyperpigmented skin areas or vascular malformations.

Other helpful data may include radiography to detect vertebral or other bony anomalies, abdominal ultrasound examinations for absent or malformed kidneys, a CT scan of brain for CNS malformations, and hematologic studies for evidence of anemia and thrombocytopenia.

Once all the data are gathered and the examination is complete, it is sometimes possible to identify a single unifying lesion (e.g., trisomy 13, 18, 21, amniotic band-induced deformations, fetal hydantoin syndrome) that may have several external manifestations. Often, however, this is not possible, and diagnosis and prognosis remain in some doubt.

ADDITIONAL COMMENTS

The presence and degree of abnormalities of the face, especially the mid-face, may give a clue to the likelihood of abnormal brain and especially forebrain development. The latter should progress normally for normal facial development to occur.

There is a danger that in labeling children with significant abnormalities in organ development, the physician will assume the task is completed, when in fact it has just begun. The physical, emotional, and social consequences for the child and his family can be severe and require empathy, patience, consistency, and understanding from the physician.

REFERENCES

1. Shepard TH: Catalog of Teratogenic Agents. Baltimore, Johns Hopkins University Press, 1975.
2. Smith, DW: Recognizable Patterns of Human Malformation. 3rd ed. Philadelphia, Saunders, 1980.
3. Warkany, J: Congenital Malformations. Chicago, Year Book, 1971.

7

TEMPERATURE REGULATION

GENERAL CONSIDERATIONS

Newborns are inefficient homeotherms. They attempt to maintain a constant body temperature, but their mechanisms for doing so can be easily overwhelmed. Heat loss occurs because of:

1. *Evaporation* (leaving a baby wet or in contact with a wet surface).
2. *Conduction* (baby in direct skin contact with a cool surface such as an unwarmed mattress).
3. *Convection* (air currents blowing over the baby such as the cool, relatively dry drafts in a delivery room).
4. *Radiation* (baby radiates heat to a cooler surface not directly in contact with the infant).

Of these, radiation is the most difficult to control. It can account for large heat losses and, ultimately, hypothermia.

Premature infants are more susceptible to heat loss because they have smaller subcutaneous stores of insulating fat; a smaller mass-to-body surface ratio, enhancing heat loss; a more open and exposed resting posture allowing more surface convective and radiative losses; and an immature temperature regulation mechanism.

All newborns will have decreased response to cold stress if they are hypoxic. Newborns do not have a capacity to shiver (increased muscle activity to generate heat) but must depend on "nonshivering thermogenesis" and on blood flow regulation to the skin to conserve heat.

MAINTAINING THE INFANT IN A NEUTRAL THERMAL ENVIRONMENT

Neutral thermal environment (NTE) is defined as the ambient temperature range in which an infant utilizes the fewest calories (least energy expenditure) to maintain a normal and constant core temperature. The temperature range will vary with size and with both postnatal and postconceptional age (see Table 7–1).

Complications of Inappropriate Thermal Environments

Excess caloric use for metabolic purposes to combat *hypothermia* limits growth, because fewer calories are available for

Table 7–1. NEUTRAL THERMAL ENVIRONMENTAL TEMPERATURES*

AGE AND WEIGHT	TEMPERATURE Starting °C	°F	Range °C
0–6 hours			
under 1200 g	35.0	95.0	34.0–35.4
1201–1500 g	34.1	93.4	33.9–34.4
1501–2500 g	33.4	92.1	32.8–33.8
over 2500 g (and more than 36 weeks)	32.9	91.2	32.0–33.8
6–12 hours			
under 1200 g	35.0	95.0	34.0–35.4
1201–1500 g	34.0	93.2	33.5–34.4
1501–2500 g	33.1	91.6	32.2–33.8
over 2500 g (and more than 36 weeks)	32.8	91.0	31.4–33.8
12–24 hours			
under 1200 g	34.0	93.2	34.0–35.4
1201–1500 g	33.8	92.8	33.3–34.3
1501–2500 g	32.8	91.0	31.8–33.8
over 2500 g (and more than 36 weeks)	32.4	90.3	31.0–33.7
24–36 hours			
under 1200 g	34.0	93.2	34.0–35.0
1201–1500 g	33.6	92.5	33.1–34.2
1501–2500 g	32.6	90.7	31.6–33.6
over 2500 g (and more than 36 weeks)	32.1	89.8	30.7–33.5

*Table reproduced with permission of Dr. Marshall Klaus. From Klaus M, Fanaroff A: Care of the High Risk Neonate. 2nd ed. Philadelphia, Saunders, 1979, pp. 102–103.

growth. Disseminated intravascular coagulation (DIC) resulting in hemorrhagic disorders may occur in severely hypothermic infants.

Hyperthermia is associated with apnea. If hyperthermia is severe, "heat stroke" may occur, with permanent brain damage and death.

Hypothermia may be a sign of sepsis. Hyperthermia, which is less common, suggests CNS abnormality, especially meningitis. A common clinical problem is deciding if temperature fluctuation in an infant represents a warning sign of serious underlying illness such as sepsis. A large gradient between peripheral temperature and core temperature is suggestive of sepsis, as is any core temperature fluctuation of greater than 1.5 degrees C over several hours.

Preventive Measures

1. Keep infants out of drafts and keep them dry.
2. Cover the head with a bonnet to lessen radiant heat loss.
3. A double-walled incubator offers advantages for smaller babies. A clear plastic shield around the baby in a single-walled incubator will also work well.
4. Maintain high (50%) relative humidity in the incubator (diminishes evaporative loss).
5. Special precautions are needed when the infant is bathed, weighed, transported, or removed from the incubator for brief periods.
6. Cold oxygen blown over the face can alter the infant's temperature.
7. Insensible water loss and basal metabolic rate are greater for infants nursed on an open overhead radiant heating table. Infants so nursed may also be at risk for person-to-person spread of infections from the people who handle them.

ADDITIONAL COMMENTS

Adequate attention to thermal needs and elimination of excessive heat loss are the first priorities of newborn care. They must precede and complement all other aspects of care.

Servo-controlled incubators and warming tables have become popular in recent years. It is critical that all the staff understand that these devices work to maintain a constant infant temperature and that fluctuation in the power output of the warming device may indicate temperature instability in the infant.

REFERENCES

1. Perlstein P, Hersh C, Glueck C, Sutherland J: Adaptation to cold in the first three days of life. Pediatrics 54:411, 1974.
2. Scopes J: Thermoregulation in the Newborn. *In* Avery, GB (ed): Neonatology: Pathophysiology and Management of the Newborn. 2nd ed. Philadelphia, Lippincott, 1981, p. 171.
3. Voora S, Srinivasan G, Lilien L, Yeh T, Pildes R: Fever in full term newborns in the first four days of life. Pediatrics 69:40, 1982.

8

NUTRITION AND FLUID ADMINISTRATION

NEONATAL NUTRITION

by Mary J. O'Leary, M.S., R.D.

GENERAL CONSIDERATIONS

1. Birth represents a major change in the source and type of nutrition for all infants, and thus presents a physiologic challenge to the premature infant.
2. Energy reserves in the low birth weight (LBW) baby are small. At 1000 g, the fetal body contains about 1% fat, compared with 16% at term (3500 g). Glycogen stores are minimal.
3. Endogenous stores of fat and protein ultimately determine the survival time of an undernourished infant.
4. Survival time can be estimated by assuming depletion of all glycogen and fat and about ⅓ of body protein tissue at a rate of 50 kcals/kg/day with 75 cc/kg/day of intravenous fluid or D10W (Table 8–1).

Table 8–1. DEPLETION TIME (DAYS)

BIRTH WEIGHT	IV FLUIDS	D10W
1000 g	4	11
2000 g	12	30
3500 g	32	80

5. The LBW infant is particularly vulnerable to undernutrition that will adversely affect his response to acute and chronic illness, his recovery time, and perhaps his long term outcome.

NUTRITIONAL REQUIREMENTS

Immediate. Water, electrolytes, and energy (glucose).

After Several Days. Protein, essential fatty acids, vitamins, and minerals.

Table 8–2. CALORIC NEEDS (LBW INFANTS)

	KCAL/KG/DAY
Basal metabolic rate	50
Activity	15
Cold stress	10
Total Maintenance	75 (range 60–80)
Specific dynamic action	8
Fecal loss	12
Growth	25
Total Additional Requirements	45
Total Caloric Needs for Growth	120 (range 105–125)

Caloric Requirements—Low Birth Weight Infants

Energy requirements may be increased by stress, metabolic mass (SGA), or growth. They may decrease in a neutral thermal environment or when absorptive loss is eliminated with parenteral nutrition (Table 8–2).

Assessment of Needs

The guidelines in Table 8–3 are suggested, recognizing that they represent minimal rather than optimal nutritional needs. Low birth weight infants who are clinically stable will meet these nutritional recommendations sooner than infants who are ill.

Protein Requirements

1. There is controversy regarding the protein requirements of the low birth weight infant. If an in utero accretion rate of protein tissue is the goal, then advisable intakes for 1000 and 1500 g infants are 3.5 and 4.0 g/kg/day, respectively. It is argued, however, that in utero growth rate is an unrealistic goal for the prematurely born infant, who no longer has the distinct nutritional advantages of the maternal-fetal connection.
2. The type of protein may be important in defining quantitative requirements. Adequate growth can occur with a whey predominant protein intake of 2 g/kg/day. The infant gains in weight and length, although more slowly than in utero rates.
3. The type of protein also affects tolerance. Casein predominant proteins (whey:casein 18:82, as in cow's milk and most standard infant formulas) are poorly tolerated by low birth weight infants. Metabolic acidosis and elevated blood levels of ammonia, and the amino acids phenylalanine and tyrosine may

Table 8–3. ASSESSMENT GUIDELINES

DAY 5

If total calorie intake is less than 60 kcals/kg/day parenteral or 80 kcal/kg/day enteral, consider these options:

1. If there are still *no enteral feedings,* consider:
   a. Peripheral vein alimentation fluids (glucose, amino acids, vitamins, and minerals), if further enteral limitation is anticipated.
   b. Central vein alimentation fluids, if prolonged enteral limitation is expected, or if poor peripheral vessel access exists. Certain surgical or GI problems, e.g., gastroschisis, may require central hyperalimentation beginning earlier.
2. If there is *poor tolerance of enteral feedings,* consider:
   a. Change in method or frequency of feeding.
   b. Change in type or concentration of feeding.

DAY 7

1. The infant should be receiving an enteral and/or parenteral source of glucose, amino acids, essential fatty acids, vitamins, and minerals (as tolerated).
2. Low weight should be reached between 4–7 days of life and should not exceed 15% reduction in birth weight (depending upon gestational age).

DAY 10

If there is no actual weight gain, or if caloric intake is less than 80 kcal/kg/day (parenteral) or 100 kcals/kg/day (enteral), consider options to increase caloric intake, e.g., increase volume and/or concentration of feeding.

DAY 14

Total caloric intake should meet infant's needs for sustained growth, i.e., 110–120 kcals/kg/day. (Note: higher caloric intakes may be needed by infants with elevated needs, e.g., SGA, chronic lung disease.)

---

occur in the neonatal period. Lactobezoars have been associated with casein predominant formulas. Whey predominant proteins (whey:casein 60:40, as in human milk and the new premature formulas) are well tolerated without these metabolic consequences.

4. Whey predominant proteins provide adequate amounts of the amino acids essential for premature infants—histidine, cystine, and tyrosine—as well as the amino acids required by mature individuals. LBW infants may also be dependent on a dietary intake of taurine, an amino sulfonic acid.
5. Protein should constitute 6–17% of calories. Less than 7% may limit growth; more than 16% may be toxic, with consequent azotemia and acidosis.

Fat

1. A major source of energy: 9 kcals/g of fat with minimal contribution to renal solute load and GI osmolality.
2. Fat should constitute 30–55% of calories. More than 60% may lead to ketosis.
3. Linoleic acid and arachidonic acid (unsaturated) are essential fatty acids (EFA). Since linoleic is converted to arachidonic acid in vivo, linoleic acid as 3–4% of total calories will prevent EFA deficiency. EFA accounts for about 7% of total calories in human milk.

4. There is poor absorption of long chain fatty acids in LBW infants owing to low intraluminal bile salt concentration and pancreatic lipase deficiency.
5. Fats containing polyunsaturated fatty acids (PUFA) are absorbed better than saturated fats. Human milk fat is well absorbed owing to the presence of lipase and other factors in human milk.
6. Medium-chain fatty acids are absorbed directly into the hepatic circulation and are not dependent on solubilization by bile salt micelles. Hence, medium-chain triglycerides (MCT) are well absorbed by LBW infants, resulting in increased weight gain, enhanced calcium absorption, and improved nitrogen retention.

Carbohydrate

1. A major source of energy. Enzymes for endogenous production of glucose from carbohydrates, proteins, and to a lesser extent fats are present in the LBW infant.
2. Carbohydrates should constitute 35–65% of calories. Too little carbohydrate may lead to hypoglycemia; too much carbohydrate may provoke loose stools.
3. Lactose is found in human and cow's milk. It supplies most or all of the carbohydrate in milk-based formulas.
4. Although lactase matures late in gestation, enzyme activity increases rapidly after birth, even in LBW infants. However, lactase is easily diminished by injury to the mucosal brush border, and secondary lactose intolerance may develop.
5. Other carbohydrate sources in proprietary formulas include sucrose and glucose, which are well absorbed and metabolized by LBW infants. Glucose polymers appear to be well tolerated but need further investigation for use in LBW infants.

Minerals

Electrolytes

Table 8–4. ELECTROLYTE REQUIREMENTS

DAILY REQUIREMENTS	MEQ/KG/DAY
Na^+	2–3
Cl^-	2
K^+	2

LBW infants may become sodium-depleted owing to renal immaturity and prolonged small volume feedings. Daily sodium intakes of 3–6 mEq or more per kg may be required by some infants to avoid hyponatremia.

Calcium and Phosphorus Requirements

1. Two-thirds of the mineral content of the body of the full term neonate is accumulated in the last trimester of pregnancy. The infant born prematurely is deprived of this important in utero mineral deposition.
2. The calcium content of human milk (35 mg/100 mL) and standard infant formula (55 mg/100 mL) is less than that needed to meet in utero calcium accretion rates (130–150 mg/kg/day). This problem is exacerbated by mineral retention rates, which are less than intake levels (as low as 50–60% of intake).
3. Growing LBW infants, especially those less than 1500 g, are at risk for developing osteoporotic bone changes and poor linear growth.
4. Supplemental calcium should be added to prevent inadequate skeletal mineralization. Optimal intake of phosphorus is unknown; however, it is recommended that phosphorus be supplemented to provide a Ca:P ratio of about 2:1, i.e., similar to that in human milk.
5. Some of the new premature formulas—e.g., Similac Special Care (Ross) and Enfamil Premature (Mead Johnson)—are already fortified with sufficient calcium and phosphorus to meet in utero accretion rates. When using these formulas, no supplementation is necessary.

Iron

1. Iron stores of premature infants begin to decrease at 2 months of age. (This decrease occurs at 4 months of age in term babies.) LBW babies may develop iron deficiency anemia by 3 months of age if supplemental iron is not given.
2. For *premature* infants, administer 2 mg iron/kg/day beginning at 8 weeks of age and/or when birth weight has doubled (Table 8–5). Iron-fortified formula at a volume and caloric intake sufficient for growth usually provides this amount of iron. If non-iron-fortified formula or breast milk is fed, supplemental iron should be given.
3. Possible negative effects of earlier iron supplementation include interference with intestinal absorption of vitamin E, intensification of the hemolytic process related to vitamin E deficiency, and interference with the antibacterial properties of transferrin and lactoferrin as they become iron-saturated (Table 8–5).

Table 8–5. IRON SUPPLEMENTATION IN INFANTS

	PRETERM	TERM
IRON SUPPLEMENT	2 mg/kg/day by 2 months	1 mg/kg/day by 4 months

Trace Minerals

Specific estimates of trace mineral requirements for full term or preterm infants are not available. The American Academy of Pediatrics (AAP) suggests intakes for premature infants based tentatively on the concentrations per 100 kcal recommended to prevent overt deficiency in full term infants (Table 8–6).

Table 8–6. ADVISABLE INTAKES OF TRACE MINERALS (PER 100 KCAL)

Zinc	0.5 mg
Copper	60 mcg
Manganese	5 mcg
Iodine	5 mcg

The need for fluoride supplementation in LBW infants is unknown.

Vitamin Requirements

1. Vitamin requirements for preterm and term infants are not precisely known. Advisable intakes have been set in excess of the estimated requirements in order to allow a margin of safety (Table 8–7).
2. Although human milk and formulas contain vitamins, neonates (LBW infants in particular) consume such small volumes that total daily vitamin intake usually falls well below advisable intake levels. Type, quantity, and frequency of vitamin supplementation varies with individual body weight and predominant feeding (Table 8–8).
3. Vitamin supplementation should be delayed until the infant has tolerated full-strength formula or breast milk for at least 48 hours, at a volume sufficient to provide calories for maintenance and growth (greater than 80 kcal/kg/day). Because common vitamin preparations have very high osmolalities, it is suggested that the supplements be mixed with the enteral feedings. This minimizes the adverse side effects of vitamin supplementation, such as increased gastric residuals and regurgitation.

Human Milk

All healthy women should be encouraged to breast feed their full term infants. The nutritional adequacy of breast milk for small premature infants is, however, a controversial subject. There is a lack of adequate data concerning the qualitative and quantitative composition of human milk, a lack of agreement regarding opti-

Table 8–7. COMPOSITION OF VITAMIN SUPPLEMENTS COMPARED TO ADVISABLE INTAKES

	ADVISABLE INTAKES		ORAL SUPPLEMENTATION	
VITAMIN	Preterm	Full Term (0–12 mos)	Polyvisol (1 cc)	Hospital-Prepared Solution of Vitamins*
Vitamin A (IU) per day	500	500	1500	1500
Vitamin D (IU)	600	400	400	400
Vitamin E (IU)	30	4	5	30
Vitamin K (mcg)	15	15	—†	—†
Vitamin C (mg)	60	20	35	60
Thiamine (mg)	0.2	0.2	0.5	0.5
Riboflavin (mg)	0.4	0.4	0.6	0.6
Niacin (mg)	5	5	8	8
B_6 (mg)	0.4	0.4	0.4	0.4
B_{12} (mcg)	1.5		2	2
Folic acid (mcg)	60	50	—	60
Pantothenic acid (mg)	2		—	3.7
Biotin (mcg)	12		—	20

*In-house preparation used on our unit based on Ziegler's advisable intakes for prematures.

†Vitamin K should be given separately; 0.5 to 1 mg IM at birth (prn thereafter) to prevent vitamin K deficiency or hemorrhagic disease of the newborn.

Table 8–8. SUGGESTED SCHEDULE FOR VITAMIN/MINERAL SUPPLEMENTATION BASED ON BODY WEIGHT AND PREDOMINANT FEEDING

	Human Milk	Similac Special Care (Ross)	Enfamil Premature (Mead Johnson), Premie SMA (Wyeth)	Similac Enfamil SMA
<2000 G INFANT				
Premie vitamins* 0.6 mL tid	yes	no	yes	yes
Vitamin D (as D_3) 400 IU/day	no	yes	no	no
Vitamin E/folate 30 IU/50 mcg/day	no	yes	no	no
Calcium (as gluceptate) 0.5–1.5mL/kg/day = 9–27 mg C^{++}/kg/day	yes	no	no	yes
Phosphorus (as potassium phosphate) 0.2mL/kg/day = 18 mg P/kg/day	yes	no	no	yes
Iron 2 mg/kg/day	Prematures: Yes, when body weight has doubled and/or infant is 8 weeks of age. No, if receiving formula with iron.			
>2000 G INFANT:				
Polyvisol 1.0 mL/day†	yes	Not usually fed to infants >2000 g		yes
Iron 1 mg/kg/day	Full term: Yes, by 4 months of age. No, if receiving formula with iron.			

*In-house preparation based on Ziegler's advisable intakes for prematures. See previous table for exact composition.

†Infants who weigh >2500 g and take about 500 mL/day receive 0.5 mL/day.

mal growth and protein requirements of LBW infants, and some difficulty in performing and interpreting clinical nutrition studies of premature infants. We feed LBW infants their own mother's milk as available, recognizing the following features and limitations of human milk composition.

1. The composition of human milk for mothers delivering prematurely apparently differs from that of mothers delivering at term. Preterm human milk contains more energy, protein, sodium, and chloride than either term or mature human milk, and it better meets the elevated nutrient needs of the LBW infant. The concentrations of these nutrients decrease with progressing lactation and approximate the levels of mature human milk at about 1 mo lactation.
2. The caloric density of preterm human milk is approximately 22 kcal/oz (i.e., 0.73 kcal/mL). Human milk fat is more concentrated in hind milk than in fore milk; therefore it is important that the breasts be fully emptied during feeding.
3. The protein in human milk is 60% whey (lactalbumin and 3-lactoglobulin) and 40% casein. Intragastrically, this whey predominant protein forms a small, flocculent curd that is easily

digested. Protein provides about 7% of total calories in human milk. This protein is of high biological value and provides adequate amounts of the amino acids that are essential for the enzymatically immature infant.

4. Fat provides 50–55% of the total calories in human milk. This fat is well absorbed, even by LBW infants, owing to the high lipolytic activity of the lipase present in human milk and the high concentration of polyunsaturated fatty acids (e.g., oleic acid).
5. Lactose is the principal carbohydrate in human milk. The concentration of lactose in preterm mothers' milk gradually increases during the first month of lactation. Although lactase matures late in gestation, lactose is usually digested well by the premature infant.
6. The concentrations of calcium and phosphorus are similar in preterm and full term human milk. Human milk does *not* meet the calcium and phosphorus needs for normal bone mineralization of infants born prematurely; supplements are recommended according to the schedule outlined in Table 8–8. Although the sodium content of preterm human milk is higher than that of full term milk, LBW infants consuming small daily volumes of human milk may become sodium-depleted; the sodium status of these infants should be monitored. Multivitamin supplementation is required following the schedule in Table 8–8.
7. Human milk contains a number of antimicrobial components that cannot be mimicked in proprietary infant formulas (e.g., immunoglobulins, leukocytes, lactoferrin, C_3, and lysozymes). Although not all of these factors have been proved effective in local or systemic immunity for the newborn, it appears that the incidence of infection and possibly necrotizing enterocolitis may be less in human milk-fed infants. Common milk storage procedures may alter the antimicrobial quality of human milk.

Proprietary Formulas

Infant formulas are usually designed to approximate the composition of human milk. Table 8–9 shows the composition of some commonly available formulas and human milk.

CHOICE OF FEEDING

Appropriate diets for infants in our intensive care nurseries are chosen using the following guidelines. These recommendations are adequate for most infants. Babies with certain GI, surgical, or other serious medical problems may require specialized formulas beyond the scope of this chapter.

Table 8–9. COMPOSITION OF HUMAN MILK AND SOME INFANT FORMULAS

	CALORIC DENSITY	PROTEIN	PROTEIN % TOTAL CALORIES	CARBOHYDRATE	CARBOHYDRATE % TOTAL CALORIES	FAT	FAT % TOTAL CALORIES	CA (MG/L)	P (MG/L)	APPROXIMATE SOLUTE LOAD (MOSM/L) Renal	GI	COMMENTS
Human Milk												
Mature	20 kcal/oz (.67 kcal/cc)	whey/casein 60:40	7	lactose	38	human milk fat	55	340	169	75	300	"State of the art" infant feeding is higher in specific nutrients than mature human milk, low in Ca^{++} and $PO_4^{=}$.
Premature	22 kcal/oz (.73 kcal/cc)	60:40		lactose		human milk fat		293	134		300	
Formulas												
Standard												
Similac Enfamil	20 kcal/oz	18:82	9	lactose	41–43	coconut and soy oils	48–50	510 520	390 438	110–120	285	Not recommended for LBW infants <1800–2000 g; meets nutrient needs and promotes normal growth in infants >2000 g.
Humanized												
SMA Similac PM 60/40	20 kcal/oz	60:40	9	lactose	43	corn, coconut, and/or soy, oleo, safflower oils	48	420 400	310 200	105 90	250 260	Demineralized whey predominant formulas that may be beneficial as initial feedings for very LBW, stressed infants. Should not be fed to growing LBW infants for prolonged periods of time, because of low protein and mineral content.

Table continued on following page

Table 8–9. COMPOSITION OF HUMAN MILK AND SOME INFANT FORMULAS (*Continued*)

	CALORIC DENSITY	PRO-TEIN	PROTEIN % TOTAL CALORIES	CARBO-HYDRATE	CARBO-HYDRATE % TOTAL CALORIES	FAT	FAT % TOTAL CALORIES	CA (MG/L)	P (MG/L)	APPROXIMATE SOLUTE LOAD (MOSM/L)		COMMENTS
										Renal	GI	
Premature												
Similac Special Care	24 kcal/oz (.8 kcal/mL)	60:40	11	lactose/glucose polymers 50:50	42	MCT/corn/coconut 50:30:20	47	1440	702	208	300	See comparison of premature versus standard formula, Table 8–10.
Premature Enfamil with Whey	same	same	12	40:60	44	40:40:20	44	940	470	220	300	
Premie SMA	same	same	10	50:50	42	coconut/safflower/oleo/soy/MCT 27:25:20:18:10	48	750	400	175	268	
Soy												
Isomil	20 kcal/oz	soy isolate	12	corn syrup solids and sucrose	40	coconut/soy oils	48	700	500	126	240	Both products are iron-fortified; hence vitamin E:PUFA ratio is of particular importance for the LBW infant at risk for hemolytic anemia. The AAP recommends a minimal E:PUFA ratio of 1:1 in LBW infants.
ProSobee	same	same	12	corn syrup solids	40	soy/coconut oils 80:20	48	788	525	160	224	

Initial Feeding for Infants

During the early period of stress, weight loss, and diuresis, the following characteristics of diet may be advantageous when initiating enteral nutrition:

1. Low renal solute load (low protein, low mineral).
2. GI osmolality ≃300 mOsm/L.
3. Protein with whey:casein ratio of 60:40.
4. Nutrient composition that is readily digestible and absorbable.
5. *Not* iron-fortified.

Feedings that meet these criteria include:

1. Preterm mother's milk.
2. Similac PM 60/40, SMA Lo-Iron.
3. Premature formula.

Note: Formula manufacturers recommend feeding premature formulas to very low birth weight infants (< 1500 g) *after* sustained weight gain is achieved. However, this frequently does not occur in these small babies until after the first week or two of postpartum life. Prior to this time, premature formulas may be diluted to half their strength (12 kcal/oz) and introduced in very small quantities. Concentration may be increased to 24 kcal/oz during the first 12–24 hours of enteral feeding, with a subsequent gradual increase in volume over several days.

Subsequent Feeding for Infants

After the initial period of stress and weight loss, when an infant is tolerating an enteral volume of 120–150 mL/kg/day, the following feeding choices are appropriate:

1. Preterm mother's milk (all weights).
2. Premature formula (<1800–2000 g body weight).
3. Standard formula (>1800–2000 g body weight).

Note: Partial formula feedings may be needed for optimal growth if human milk volume is limited to <150 mL/kg/day.

Table 8–10 shows the compositional differences between premature and standard formulas and lists the advantages in choosing premature formulas for preterm infants.

A lactose-free soy protein isolate formula is sometimes used to feed newborn infants. The specific indications for its use are sensitivity to cow milk protein, postdiarrheal lactase deficiency, and other disorders causing lactose intolerance. Very LBW infants fed lactose-free soy protein formula apparently *do* adequately utilize soy protein (as documented by nitrogen retention rates similar to fetal accretion rates) and *do not* experience a deleterious effect on calcium retention or homeostasis related to the absence of lactose. However, phosphorus absorption is diminished with the feeding of soy formula and may, over time, strain phosphorus homeostatic control mechanisms. If feeding lactose-free soy protein formula is indicated for VLBW infants (e.g., in cases of lac-

Table 8–10. COMPARISON OF PREMATURE VERSUS STANDARD FORMULAS FOR FEEDING PRETERM INFANTS

PREMATURE FORMULAS*	STANDARD FORMULAS†
1. Designed, tested in preterm infants.	1. Designed, tested in term infants.
2. *Protein:* Whey:casein 60:40.	2. Whey:casein 18:82.
3. *Carbohydrate:* 50% lactose, 50% glucose polymers. (Note: This carbohydrate blend helps keep osmolality of formulas within isotonic range.)	3. 100% lactose. (Note: This is well tolerated by most prematures.)
4. *Fat:* Part medium-chain triglycerides, part long-chain fats (which provide essential fatty acids). a. Similac Special Care: 50% MCT, 92% total fat absorption. b. Premature Enfamil with Whey: 50% MCT, 93% total fat absorption. c. Premie SMA: 10% MCT, total fat absorption unknown.	4. 100% long-chain fats.
5. *24 kcal/oz:* Growth needs better met within fluid tolerance ranges. 150 mL/kg/day to provide 120 kcal/kg/day.	5. *20 kcal/oz:* 180 mL/kg/day to provide 120 kcal/kg/day.
6. *Calcium/Phosphorus* a. Similac Special Care: No supplementation needed to meet 3rd trimester fetal accretion rates. b. Premature Enfamil with Whey: No supplementation needed. c. Premie SGA: Partial supplementation may be desirable.	6. Calcium/Phosphorus-fortified to meet the requirements of term infants; additional supplements needed for preterm infants.
7. *Vitamins* a. Similac Special Care: Vitamin D, E. Folate supplements may be needed. b. Premature Enfamil with Whey: Multivitamin supplement needed. c. Premie SMA: Multivitamin supplement needed.	7. Vitamin-fortified to meet term infant needs; multivitamin supplement needed for preterm infants.

*Similac Special Care (Ross), Enfamil Premature (Mead Johnson), Premie SMA (Wyeth).

†Similac (20 kcal/oz), Enfamil (20 kcal/oz).

Table 8–11. USE OF LACTOSE-FREE SOY PROTEIN FORMULA IN PREMATURE INFANTS*

FEED ISOMIL	
Short term diarrhea	10–14 days
Long term diarrhea	>450 g weight gain

*All soy formula products are currently iron-fortified; hence, the vitamin E:polyunsaturated fatty acid ratio (E:PUFA) is of particular importance for the LBW infant at risk for hemolytic anemia. The American Academy of Pediatrics recommends a minimum E:PUFA ratio of 1:1 in LBW infants.

tase deficiency or lactose intolerance), the schedule in Table 8–11 should be followed. If extended use of this formula is required (e.g., in cases of cow milk protein sensitivity), the infant should be monitored for potential adverse effects on skeletal mineralization.

Caloric Supplements

MCT (medium chain triglyceride) oil (Mead Johnson) and Polycose (Ross) are dietary supplements that increase caloric density without marked alterations in mineral content or solute load. Both supplements alter the relative distribution of total calories between protein, carbohydrates, and fat. Because even small amounts of MCT oil or Polycose reduce the percentage of calories as protein while altering the percentage of calories as fat and carbohydrate, we do *not* add these supplements to human milk or standard 20 kcal/oz formulas (see Table 8–12).

Table 8–12. POTENTIAL ADVERSE EFFECTS OF MCT OIL AND POLYCOSE SUPPLEMENTS IN HUMAN MILK AND STANDARD 20 KCAL/OZ FORMULA

	PERCENT DISTRIBUTION OF CALORIES AS		
	PROTEIN	CARBOHYDRATE	FAT
Human Milk	7	38	55
(150 mL/day)			
+0.4 mL MCT/oz	5 (low)	33 (low)	63 (high)
+1.5 mL PC/oz	3–4 (low)	38	60 (high)
Standard Formula*	9	42	49
(150 mL/day)			
+0.4 mL MCT/oz	7	35 (low)	57
+1.5 mL PC/oz	6 (low)	43	50

*Standard formula as Similac (20) or Enfamil (20).

If it is necessary to increase the caloric concentration of feedings (if infant is gaining <1–2% body weight per day on >120 kcal/kg/day *and* if maximum volume is reached), add MCT and then Polycose to either premature formula or concentrated standard formula up to a maximum of 60% of total calories as fat and a minimum of 7% of total calories as protein. Specifically, take a 24 kcal/oz formula base, add 0.4 cc MCT oil/oz (= 27 kcal/oz formula), and then add 1.5 mL liquid Polycose/oz (=30 kcal/oz formula). Increase the volume of feeding as tolerated, and wean off MCT oil and Polycose as soon as possible.

ADDITIONAL COMMENTS

Nutritional standards based on proven data are insufficient for the LBW infant. These recommendations attempt to strike a balance in areas where there is disagreement or controversy. New data and products will undoubtedly emerge in the future.

REFERENCES

1. Avery GB, Fletcher AB: Nutrition. *In* Avery GB (ed): Neonatology: Pathophysiology and Management of the Newborn. Philadelphia, Lippincott, 1981.
2. Committee on Nutrition, American Academy of Pediatrics: Nutritional needs of low birth weight infants. Pediatrics 60:519, 1977.
3. Lebenthal E (ed): Textbook of Gastroenterology and Nutrition in Infancy. New York, Raven Press, 1981, vols. 1 and 2.
4. Brady MS, et al: Formulas and human milk for premature infants: A review and update. J Amer Diet Assoc 81:547, 1982.
5. Ziegler EE, Biga RL, Fomon SJ: Nutritional requirements of the premature infant. *In* Suskind RM (ed): Textbook of Pediatric Nutrition. New York, Raven Press, 1981.

FLUID AND GLUCOSE ADMINISTRATION

GENERAL CONSIDERATIONS

1. Management of nearly all sick infants, whether term or preterm, involves intravenous fluid administration. It is imperative to understand the wide range of factors affecting the physiology of water balance, including gestational age, postnatal age, appropriateness of weight for gestational age, thermal stress, and clinical conditions.
2. Fluid therapy is intimately related to nutrition.
3. Consider body composition:

Table 8–13. BODY COMPOSITION

	LBW INFANT	FULL TERM
Total Body Water (TBW)	85–90%	80%
Extracellular Fluid (ECF)	50–55%	45%

4. Homeostatic mechanisms:
   a. Antidiuretic hormone (ADH) and aldosterone mechanisms intact in LBW infant.
   b. Neonatal renal function:
      i. Low glomerular filtration rate.
      ii. Obligatory Na loss.
      iii. Impaired concentrating ability (maximum 700–800 mOsm/L).
      iv. Compromised net acid excretion.
5. There is a relatively large insensible water loss owing to the large surface area/body weight ratio, increased skin permeability, and increased respiratory rate.

6. Fluid overload may lead to cardiopulmonary compromise and metabolic complications.

FLUID THERAPY

1. Estimate daily water requirements:

Table 8–14. DAILY WATER REQUIREMENTS

	ML/100 KCAL	ML/KG/DAY
Urine	50–100	60–125(2.5–5.2/kg/hr)
Insensible Water Loss	30–50	37–60
Stool	10	10–15
Sweat	0	0
Oxidation	−12	−15
Growth	+12	+15
	90–160	107–200(1–1.5 mL/kcal)

2. Total daily fluid administration is generally increased by 10–15 mL/kg/day, depending on urine output, estimate of insensible loss, and clinical status.

Table 8–15. GUIDELINES FOR FLUID INTAKE

	(ML/KG/DAY D10W)	
	<1000 G	>1500 G
Day 1	100	70
Daily increment	10–20	10–15
Day 4–5	150±20	130±20

3. Urine output is a major portion of water loss.
   a. Normal output is 2–5 mL/kg/hr.
   b. Specific gravity usually 1.005–1.010.
   c. Osmolarity usually ±250 mOsm/L.
4. Estimate insensible water loss—inversely proportional to gestational age. Evaporative water loss dissipates 25% of calories.
   a. Increased insensible water loss:
      i. Phototherapy +50%.
      ii. Radiant warmer +50%.
      iii. Single-walled incubator.
      iv. Respiratory distress (tachypnea).
      v. Temperature above thermal neutrality (+100–200%).
      vi. Core temperature elevated (+100–200%).
      vii. Sweating impaired in infants >36 weeks' and absent in infants <30 weeks' gestation.

b. Decreased insensible loss:
   i. Heat shields (−25%).
   ii. Thermal blanket—silver swaddler (−70%).
   iii. Sheep skin placed underneath the baby.
   iv. Increased environmental humidity.
   v. Heated humidified inspired air.

5. Oliguria for 1–3 days often occurs in infants with hyaline membrane disease, asphyxia, and inappropriate ADH secretion. Fluids should be restricted if cerebral edema is suspected (asphyxia, seizures).
6. Monitor:
   a. Intake, hourly.
   b. Output, hourly.
   c. Body weight, daily (expect 10 g/kg/day loss for 5–10 days).
   d. Urine specific gravity (SG) or osmolarity, q 8 hr.
   e. Urine glucose.
   f. Serum Na^+, K^+, BUN (blood urea nitrogen), daily.
   g. Temperature, q 2–4 hr.
   h. Blood pressure, q 1–4 hr or continuously.
   i. Peripheral circulatory status, edema.
   j. Mucous membrane moisture and skin turgor.
7. Increased risk of patent ductus arteriosus (PDA) exists if daily fluid exceeds 180 mL/kg/day; however, fluid intake must depend on the magnitude of water losses.

INTRAVENOUS GLUCOSE

1. Initial infusion of D10W will prevent hypoglycemia and spare tissue protein breakdown.
2. Optimum is 8–9 g/kg/day, since glucose is assimilated at about 6 mg/kg/min.
3. Calculate glucose load: g glucose/mL × mL/unit time.
4. Caloric content and osmolarity:

Table 8–16. CALORIC CONTENT AND OSMOLARITY

DEXTROSE/WATER	KCAL/ML	MOSM/L
5%	0.17	252
7.5%	0.25	378
10%	0.34	505
15%	0.51	758
20%	0.68	1010

5. Monitor:
   a. Urine glucose, q 8 hr.
   b. Serum glucose, daily.
   c. Dextrostix or Chemstrip, q 8 hr or prn.

6. Wean at rate of 5 mg/dL/12 hr in the absence of hypoglycemia.

ELECTROLYTES

1. Intravenous electrolytes will depend on renal excretion rates, other losses, and catabolic state. IV electrolytes are usually delayed until second day. Active growth requires 0.5–1.0 mEq of Na^+, K^+, and Cl^-/kg/day. Renal sodium loss is greater in LBW infants than large preterm infants; it may be 5–10 mEq/day.
2. Excess sodium excretion is defined as >3mEq/kg/day.

Table 8–17. ELECTROLYTE EXCRETION GUIDELINES

	(MEQ/KG/DAY)	
	0–24 hr	24–48 hr
Na^+	2	2–3
Cl^-	2	2–3
K^+	0	1–3 (add K^+ to IV when renal function is established)
Ca^{++}	0.5	0.5–1

3. Monitor:
   a. Serum Na^+, K^+, and Cl^- daily.
   b. Urine Na^+ output if there is serum abnormality.
   c. Urine SG or osmolarity.
4. Note: Use of diuretics, theophylline, high free water load, or oliguria will alter daily supplemental needs. Use of $NaHCO_3$ or Na acetate is determined by acid-base status.

ADDITIONAL COMMENTS

1. Severity and type of disease greatly influence fluid and electrolyte therapy.
2. Degree of prematurity and birth weight in combination with clinical abnormalities dictates the unique requirements of each infant.
3. Replacement must consider abnormal electrolyte and fluid losses via gastric suction, diarrhea, chest tube drainage, ileostomy, ascites, and the cardiocirculatory system.

REFERENCES

1. Bell EF, Neidich GA, Cashore WJ, et al: Combined effect of radiant warmer and phototherapy on insensible water loss in low birth weight infant. J Pediatr 94:810, 1979.
2. Bell EF, Warburton D, Stonestreet BS, et al: Randomized trial comparing high (HV) and low-volume (LV) maintenance fluid administration in low-birth-weight-infants. Pediatr Res 13:489, 1979.
3. Uttley WS, Habel AH: Fluid and electrolyte metabolism in the newborn infant. Clin Endocrinol Metab 5:3, 1976.

PARENTERAL NUTRITION

GENERAL CONSIDERATIONS

1. Total parenteral nutrition (TPN) is defined as the intravenous administration of a hypertonic solution of amino acids, carbohydrates, fats, electrolytes, minerals, and vitamins sufficient to sustain a positive nitrogen balance.
2. Partial parenteral nutrition is defined as administration of amino acids and carbohydrates, with or without lipids, that meet part of the maintenance caloric needs or supplement enteral feedings.
3. Total parenteral nutrition generally requires the placement of a central venous catheter, whereas partial nutrition without the use of hypertonic glucose solutions can be given by peripheral vein.
4. There are a number of real and potential complications and much controversy regarding risks versus benefits. Therefore, the indications, amounts, types, timing, and routes of TPN have not been standardized.

EXAMPLES OF INDICATIONS

1. Bowel surgery (anastomoses, resection).
2. Necrotizing enterocolitis.
3. Anomalies of the gastrointestinal tract (gastroschisis, omphalocele).
4. Very LBW infants.
5. LBW infants with prolonged severe respiratory distress.
6. Poor tolerance of enteral feedings (regurgitation, malabsorption).
7. Severe prolonged diarrhea.

ROUTE

Peripheral Vein

Used for short term supplementation when peripheral venous access is good, and for administration of isotonic or hypertonic solutions.

Central Vein

Indicated for long term supplementation, total nutritional needs, poor peripheral veins, or hypertonic solutions.

Accepted sites include the jugular vein (facial vein, internal-external jugular [percutaneous cut down]), saphenous vein, and subclavian vein.

Catheter should be placed with strict aseptic technique, usually in OR under general anesthesia. Confirm catheter placement by radiograph.

Umbilical Artery

The placement of an umbilical artery catheter solely for the administration of parenteral nutrition is not warranted. Some LBW infants who require an umbilical catheter for blood gas monitoring may need short term parenteral nutrition. In this situation, the risks of infection and fluid overload with multiple catheters and the lack of sufficient peripheral vein access may make it appropriate to administer parenteral nutritional solutions through the umbilical artery cannula. Removal of the catheter should be dictated by the need for arterial blood gas monitoring.

COMPOSITION

(See section on Neonatal Nutrition, this chapter.)

1. Calories: 50% fat, 10% protein, 40% carbohydrates.
2. Water: 120–160 mL/kg.
3. Glucose: D10W = 0.34 kcal/mL and 505 mOsm/L. See Chapter 13 for other dextrose concentrations.
4. Protein: 1.5–2.5 g/kg/day.
   a. Use crystalline amino acids. Several commercial solutions are available: $1\frac{1}{16}$%, $2\frac{1}{8}$%, or $4\frac{1}{4}$%.
   b. L-cysteine is unstable and should be added to the solution just prior to use.
5. Lipid: 2–3 g/kg/day.
   a. Prevention of EFA deficiency requires at least 0.5 g/kg/day intravenous lipids.
   b. Use 10% emulsion—280 mOsm/L; fat particles are 0.4–0.5 μ in diameter.

c. Intralipid 10% is a commonly used product made up of 10% soybean oil, 1.2% egg yolk phospholipids, 2.25% glycerine and water. Fatty acid composition is linoleic 54%, oleic 26%, palmitic 9%, and linolenic 8%.
d. The rate of administration should not exceed 0.15 g/kg/hr to prevent hyperlipemia.
e. Partial parenteral nutrition to prevent EFA deficiency requires 9–10% of caloric input as fat to provide sufficient linoleic acid.

6. Minerals and electrolytes: see section on Neonatal Nutrition, this chapter.
7. Vitamins: see Table 8–18.

Table 8–18. U.S. RECOMMENDED DAILY ALLOWANCE (RDA)

Vitamin A	1500 IU
Vitamin D	400 IU
Vitamin E	5 IU (LBW infants 15–25 IU/day)
Vitamin C	35 mg
Folic Acid	0.1 mg
Thiamine	0.5 mg
Riboflavin	0.6 mg
Niacin	8 mg
Vitamin B_6	0.4 mg
Vitamin B_{12}	2 mcg
Biotin	0.05 mg
Pantothenic Acid	3 mg

8. Trace elements: see Table 8–19.

Table 8–19. TRACE ELEMENTS

	TERM	LBW
Zinc	50–100 mcg/kg	200–300 mcg/kg
Copper	20–30 mcg/kg	40–60 mcg/kg

9. Iron: not recommended for TPN solutions.

PRECAUTIONS

1. Calories may be limited by fluid tolerance.
2. Some multiple vitamin preparations do not contain folic acid (add 50–100 mcg/day) (M.V.I.–12 contains folic acid) and vitamin K (give 1 mg IM dose weekly).
3. Since calcium is provided intravenously rather than through

intestinal absorption, 200–250 IU of vitamin D/day is considered adequate.

4. No intravenous form of vitamin E is presently available—15–25 IU/day should be given orally as soon as feasible.
5. Filters should not be used with Intralipid 10%.
6. Lipid emulsions should be infused through a separate system and administered through the same vein by means of a Y-connector near the infusion site. The Y-arm of the lipid solution should be uppermost to prevent pooling.
7. Separate infusion pumps should be used for each solution.
8. Although 20% lipid emulsions are available, 10% solutions are indicated owing to a maximum rate of infusion of 0.15 g/kg/hr.
9. $NaHCO_3$ infusion may cause precipitation.
10. Maintain strict aseptic technique and laminar flow hood while mixing solutions.
11. The solution is usable for 48 hr if refrigerated but only 24 hr once entered.
12. Use an 0.22 μ filter for all but lipid infusions.

POSSIBLE COMPLICATIONS

1. Hyperglycemia.
2. Hypoglycemia—sudden cessation of infusion.
3. Electrolyte imbalance.
4. Metabolic acidosis (amino acids).
5. Azotemia.
6. Hyperammonemia (associated with infusion of protein hydrolysate).
7. Hypervitaminosis A.
8. Anemia.
9. Hepatocellular damage (rare).
10. Thrombocytopenia.
11. Increased risk of infection.
12. Hyperlipemia.
13. Impairment of pulmonary gas exchange (hyperlipemia).
14. High FFA (free fatty acid) levels may impair glucose metabolism.
15. Displacement of bilirubin from albumin by FFA.
16. Increased risk of sepsis.
17. Thrombosis of a central vein.
18. Occlusion of catheter.

MONITORING

1. Growth: weight daily, length and occipital frontal circumference (OFC) weekly.
2. Glucose: Dextrostix and urine dipstick q 8 hr. Serum glucose prn.

D10W	ml	NEONATAL RECOMMENDED DOSE/24 HOURS
D15W	ml	CALORIES 110-140 kcal/kg
D20W	ml	PROTEIN 2-3 Gm/kg (Low Birthweight - LBW)
2 1/8% CRYSTALLINE AMINO ACID	ml	1.5-2 Gm/kg (Term)
4 1/4% CRYSTALLINE AMINO ACID	ml	

WRITE FOR 24 HOUR PERIOD ONLY	THE FOLLOWING ADDITIVES ARE TO BE INCLUDED WITH SOLUTIONS		
	SOLUTION #		NEONATAL RECOMMENDED DOSE/24 HOURS
SODIUM CHLORIDE		mEq	3-4 mEq/kg
SODIUM ACETATE		mEq	
POTASSIUM CHLORIDE		mEq	2-3 mEq/kg (POTASSIUM REQUIREMENT SHOULD BE MET BY POTASSIUM PHOSPHATE.)
POTASSIUM PHOSPHATE		mEq	2-3 mEq/kg POTASSIUM (1.5-2 mM PHOSPHATE)
CALCIUM GLUCEPTATE		mEq	1-2 mEq/kg
MAGNESIUM SULFATE		mEq	0.5-1 mEq/kg
FOLIC ACID		mcg	50-100 mcg/DAY
MVI		ml	1 ml/DAY
OR VISYNERAL		ml	0.5 ml/DAY
BEROCCA - C		ml	0.5 ml/DAY
VITAMIN K		mg	1 mg/WEEK
ZINC		mcg	200-300 mcg/kg (LBW) 50-100 mcg/kg (TERM)
COPPER		mcg	40-60 mcg/kg (LBW) 20-30 mcg/kg (TERM)
OTHER			
			TPN RATE (ml/hr)
ADDITIONAL TPN ORDERS			
I.V. FAT EMULSION 10%	PLUS 30 ml FOR TUBING	ml	2-3 Gm/kg — FAT EMULSION RATE (ml/hr)
SEE UH/HMC NEONATAL TPN PROTOCOL FOR FURTHER INFORMATION, WHICH IS AVAILABLE FROM THE DEPARTMENT OF PHARMACY SERVICES.			PHYSICIAN'S SIGNATURE — DATE

PT. NO.

NAME

D.O.B.

UNIVERSITY OF WASHINGTON HOSPITALS
HARBORVIEW MEDICAL CENTER
UNIVERSITY HOSPITAL
SEATTLE, WASHINGTON

NEONATAL TOTAL PARENTERAL NUTRITION ORDERS

UH 0411 OCT 79

WHITE - MEDICAL CHART
CANARY - PHARMACY
PINK - NURSING

3. Intake and output q 8–24 hr.
4. Na^+, K^+, Cl^-, HCO_3^- daily for 7–10 days, then q o day.
5. BUN, creatinine weekly.
6. Ca, Mg, PO_4, weekly.
7. Hematocrit reading weekly.
8. Bilirubin as indicated but at least weekly.
9. Alkaline phosphatase, serum glutamic-oxaloacetic transaminase (SGOT), and serum glutamic-pyruvic transaminase (SGPT) q o week.
10. Zn, Cu q o week.
11. Prothrombin time q o week.

SUGGESTED PROTOCOL

1. See copy of physician order sheet (Fig. 8–1).
2. New orders should be written q 24 hr and 12 hr prior to start.
3. A standard volume of 250 mL is used for each solution regardless of rate of infusion.
4. Order desired dextrose concentration and protein.
   Example:

D20W	125 mL
2⅛% amino acid	125 mL
+ electrolytes	250 mL
	(10% dextrose and 1¹/₁₆% protein)

5. Determine daily fluid requirement.
6. Calculate total minerals and vitamins to be added to 250 mL.
   Example:
   1 kg infant with fluid requirement of 125 mL/kg/day.
   Nutrients are multiplied by 250/125 = 2.0.

9 RESPIRATORY DISORDERS

INTRODUCTION

Respiratory tract diseases are the most common group of life-threatening diseases in newborns. The special needs of infants with respiratory diseases have prompted the development of special care centers for newborns. Questions still remain about basic pathophysiologic mechanisms for some of these diseases, and controversies occur over optimal treatments.

Not all signs of respiratory distress include problems directly referable to the cardiorespiratory system. Severe metabolic acidosis or congenital cyanotic heart disease (see Chapter 11) can produce significant tachypnea. Similarly, seizure activity (see Chapter 15) may be mistaken for apneic or cyanotic episodes. However, the most common causes of tachypnea and labored breathing are disorders of the respiratory tract. Therefore, the following discussion focuses on respiratory disorders in the newborn.

HYALINE MEMBRANE DISEASE OR RESPIRATORY DISTRESS SYNDROME

GENERAL CONSIDERATIONS

Definition. Hyaline membrane disease (HMD) is a condition of pulmonary insufficiency beginning at or within hours of birth, with characteristic clinical, radiographic, and physiologic signs.

Etiology. The syndrome occurs because of a deficiency of surface-tension–lowering materials in the alveoli owing to inadequate synthesis, secretion from cellular sites, inappropriate inactivation possibly due to extravascular fluid exudation, or misalignment of integral components of the surfactant system.

CLINICAL CHARACTERISTICS

1. Infants at risk include premature, appropriately grown infants, especially of less than 35 weeks' gestation; infants of diabetic mothers, especially of less than 38 weeks' gestation; infants

delivered by cesarean section without prior labor; and the second-born of twins. Birth asphyxia may also potentiate risk of disease.

2. Signs of increased work of breathing (tachypnea greater than 60 breaths/min; intercostal, substernal, and infraclavicular retractions; nasal flaring) usually begin within a few minutes of birth.
3. An expiratory grunt is usually present and increases with increasing severity of the disease.
4. The natural history of HMD is variable. Many infants with uncomplicated disease have a peak in severity by 24 to 48 hr of life with gradual improvement over several days thereafter, but some may have a more protracted course of 5 to 7 days, with slower but still complete resolution. Diuresis often accompanies the clinical and pulmonary improvement. Peripheral edema, which develops during the first 48 hr (in spite of overall weight loss), also diminishes with respiratory improvement.

DIAGNOSIS

Differential diagnosis includes anatomic disorders of the respiratory tract—all of which can also occur in prematures (see section on Congenital Airway Malformations in this chapter)—and neonatal pneumonia, especially that caused by Group B streptococcal disease (see Chapter 14). A milder form of respiratory distress in newborns, so-called transient tachypnea of the newborn, may produce some of the clinical signs of HMD but has a much shorter natural history and a different radiographic appearance, with no air bronchograms. Transient tachypnea often occurs in near term infants delivered by cesarean section. (The management of transient tachypnea consists of supplemental oxygen, warmth, withholding feedings to minimize risk of aspiration, and considering other possible causes of respiratory distress.)

DIAGNOSTIC CRITERIA

1. Hyaline membrane disease is a syndrome—the clinical findings reflect the abnormal surface tension properties producing diminished lung volume stability at the end of each expiration. The tendency of the air space to collapse is overcome by increased work of breathing, which is reflected in the previously mentioned signs.
2. Diagnostic criteria include all of the following:
   a. Hypoxemia (arterial PO_2 less than 50 mm Hg in room air) because of increased venous admixture, responsive to supplemental inspired oxygen.

b. Air bronchograms and a granular lung field appearance are evident in the chest radiograph.
c. Previously described signs of labored breathing.

3. A sample of amniotic fluid obtained prior to delivery, in which the lecithin to sphingomyelin (L/S) ratio is <2, is suggestive of pulmonary immaturity and increased risk of development of HMD.

Table 9–1. HMD: RANGE OF SEVERITY

	MILD	SEVERE
Radiographic	Air bronchograms	Little aeration White-appearing lungs
Clinical	Tachypnea Retractions Grunting on expiration Alert infant	Apneic spells Increasing frequency of apnea Gasping respirations Obtundation
Blood Gas Tensions		
PaO_2	Low (less than 50 mm Hg)	Low
$PaCO_2$	Low to normal (less than 40 mm Hg)	High (more than 45 mm Hg)
pH	Compensated acidosis	Uncompensated acidosis (pH less than 7.2)

No other laboratory data are needed to diagnose HMD, although many other abnormalities may occur as the disease progresses.

THERAPY

1. At present, therapy is supportive in nature. Experimental studies are again focusing on specific treatment with introduction of synthetic or naturally derived surfactant materials into the airways at or shortly after birth.
2. Major aspects of supportive therapy are directed at supporting gas exchange. This is accomplished first by providing supplemental, warmed, humidified oxygen in sufficient concentration to maintain the arterial PaO_2 between 50 and 70 mm Hg. The application of continuous distending airway pressure via nasal prongs or an intrapharyngeal tube using pressures of 6–8 cm H_2O may aid in this, although initial enthusiasm for this treatment has diminished recently. Profound hypoxemia (PaO_2 less than 50 mm HG with F_IO_2 greater than 0.80) and/or hypercarbia ($PaCO_2$ greater than 60 mm Hg or rapidly rising toward this level) are indications for assisted ventilation (see Chapter 20).
3. Other aspects of supportive care include providing adequate warmth (see Chapter 7); adequate fluid intake with appropriate electrolytes; and adequate glucose intake to prevent or correct hypoglycemia and maintain blood glucose levels greater than 30 mg/100 mL.

Severe metabolic acidosis should be corrected with a slow infusion of sodium bicarbonate (maximum 1 mEq/min) in diluted concentration (1 mEq/2 mL fluid) to treat pH less than 7.2 with a normal $PaCO_2$. Often metabolic and respiratory acidosis coexist, and both bicarbonate and assisted ventilation will be necessary to restore acid base status to normal.

Ready access to arterial blood is critical for the management of HMD. This usually means placement of an umbilical arterial catheter. Although arterial catheters have many complications, they provide a rapid means of obtaining much physiologic information with little added disturbance of the baby. (See Chapter 20 for details of placement.) Recent evidence suggests that alterations in arterial oxygen levels may occur with any manipulation of the infant.

COMPLICATIONS OF HMD AND ITS TREATMENT

Pneumothorax (PT) occurs in 30% of mechanically ventilated newborns with HMD. PT is hazardous because it may inhibit venous cardiac return and hence cardiac output, as well as produce collapse of previously ventilated lung regions. Treatment is accomplished by inserting a No. 10 or No. 12 Fr thoracostomy tube into the pleural space. The tip of the tube should be positioned in the superior anterior pleural space. Pneumomediastinum (PMN), another form of extra-alveolar air leak, rarely requires treatment as it does not usually interfere with pulmonary func-

Table 9–2. HMD: COMPLICATIONS

PULMONARY	Acute: Air leak complications, Pulmonary interstitial emphysema (PIE), Pneumothorax (PT), Superimposed pulmonary infection, Pneumomediastinum (PMN), Pneumopericardium (PPC).
	Chronic: Chronic lung disease.
CARDIOVASCULAR	Patent ductus arteriosus (PDA), systemic hypotension.
RENAL	Oliguria.
METABOLIC	Hypo- or hypernatremia.
	Metabolic acidosis.
	Hypoglycemia.
	Starvation.
HEMATOLOGIC	Anemia (often because of excessive losses in blood tests).
	Hemorrhage, especially intracranial and/or pulmonary.
IATROGENIC	Thrombotic or embolic complication of umbilical catheter.
	Malposition of catheter with inadvertent sampling of pulmonary arterial blood resulting in excessive supplemental oxygen administration and hyperoxia.
OTHER	Retrolental fibroplasia.

tion. Other air leaks occur less commonly. (See section on Pulmonary Air Leak, this chapter, for a more detailed discussion of all air leaks.)

An important pulmonary complication of HMD and its treatment is the development of bronchopulmonary dysplasia (BPD), a discussion of which is beyond the scope of this book.

Another commonly associated complication is the development of a patent ductus arteriosus. The left-to-right shunt through the open ductus increases pulmonary blood flow, potentially causing decreased respiratory system compliance, increased work of breathing, worsened hypoxemia, and radiographic changes of increased lung density. See Chapter 11 for discussion of treatment.

Table 9–2 lists other complications.

OUTCOME

Long term developmental morbidity appears to be related to complications of prematurity other than HMD.

Table 9–3. SURVIVAL OF HMD INFANTS BY BIRTH WEIGHT*

BIRTH WEIGHT	SURVIVAL OF INFANTS WITH HMD (%)
less than 1000 g	40
1000–1250 g	72
1251–1500 g	90
1501–2000 g	92
2001–2500 g	96

*University of Washington Hospital, Seattle, Wash., Neonatal Intensive Care Unit, 1980 data.

ADDITIONAL COMMENTS

1. The risk of developing HMD can be lowered, especially in females, by antenatal maternal administration of betamethasone or dexamethasone, 24 mg administered in 2 or 3 doses over 24 hr prior to delivery. Labor-inhibiting medications, including $beta_2$-agonist drugs, may also decrease risk of HMD by direct effects on fetal pulmonary maturation, as well as by delaying delivery.
2. Care of the premature infant with moderate or severe HMD is best performed in a center capable of dealing with the complications listed and able to provide in-house round-the-clock support by physicians, nurses, respiratory therapists, and appropriate laboratory and x-ray personnel. Successful treatment of HMD has been closely associated with improvements in regionalization of care for sick newborns.

Table 9–4. SEQUENCE OF STEPS IN INITIAL MANAGEMENT OF HMD

A premature newborn with HMD imposes many demands on an often stressed medical and nursing staff. The first priority after birth for an infant at risk for HMD is:

RESUSCITATION

1. Establish an adequate airway by suctioning, positioning the infant's head, use of an oral airway, or oral intubation.
2. Assess ventilation.
3. Establish that cardiac output is adequate by monitoring the pulse rate, which should be greater than 100 beats/min and routinely greater than 140 beats/min. (See Chapter 3 on Resuscitation.)

ASSURANCE OF WARMTH

1. Dry thoroughly with a warm towel.
2. Use an extraneous heat source. *Caution:* Covering the baby with towels while he is underneath the radiant heating element on a warming table interferes with his temperature regulation.

The following steps then need to be carried out rapidly:

1. Blood gas determination, because in premature infants skin color is poorly correlated with arterial PO_2.
2. Chest radiograph to survey the extent of the disease and the early development of air leak complications.
3. Rapid diagnosis of air leak complications, which can happen very early in the course of severe HMD.

CORRECTION OF METABOLIC ABNORMALITIES

The only immediate problems are glucose and acid-base status.

Premature infants with significant respiratory distress can be presumed to have HMD and will need arterial monitoring for optimal care. We therefore suggest delaying a chest radiograph until an umbilical arterial catheter is placed so that its position and the degree of disease reflected by radiographic appearance can be detected with one radiographic procedure. Chest radiographs will determine the presence of a PT. Early placement of a catheter can also speed the controlled delivery of glucose and minimize the risk of hypoglycemia. If difficulty is encountered in obtaining arterial blood, venous blood may be used to assess pH and PCO_2, which can indicate the need for assisted ventilation and bicarbonate infusion. If arterial catheters are not routinely placed in the hospital of delivery, then establish a venous access for glucose, maintain the baby's temperature, and arrange for transport to another medical center (see Chapter 20 on Transport).

OTHER THERAPY

This may include antibiotic administration if there is any evidence from the history that the infant might be infected. A blood culture should be obtained prior to antibiotic therapy. The culture can be obtained through the umbilical catheter at the time of insertion; otherwise it should be obtained by venipuncture.

3. Care of the infant includes reassurance of the typically bewildered and frightened parents.

REFERENCES

1. Farrell P, Avery M: Hyaline membrane disease. Am Rev Resp Dis 111:657, 1975.
2. Hodson W, Guthrie R: Hyaline membrane disease. *In* Kelley VC (ed): Practice of Pediatrics. Hagerstown, Maryland, Harper and Row, 1979, vol. 1, ch. 85A.
3. Longman C, Engle W, Baumgart S, Fox W, Polin R: Diuretic phase of respiratory distress syndrome and its relationship to oxygen. J Pediatr 98:462, 1981.

MECONIUM ASPIRATION SYNDROME

GENERAL CONSIDERATIONS

Definition. Meconium, a mixture of bile salts and epithelial cells that makes up the contents of the fetal intestinal tract, can be aspirated into the lungs shortly before or at the time of delivery. Meconium aspiration may occur in a setting of severe asphyxia; therefore, infants with meconium aspiration pneumonia are at risk for hypoxia-induced developmental problems of the central nervous system. Meconium may be released into the amniotic fluid when fetal hypoxia increases intestinal peristaltic activity and relaxes sphincter tone.

Pathogenesis. Patchy bilateral airway obstruction occurs immediately after aspiration. Inflammation develops in response to inhaled material, especially bile salts, during the second 24 hr of the illness. Mild meconium aspiration (MAS) is sometimes associated with the development of the syndrome of persistent fetal circulation (see Chapter 11).

PREVENTION

The disease can sometimes be minimized by suctioning the infant's airway before effective respirations have begun. However, prolongation of this procedure can be hazardous, as the infant's overall status may worsen while prolonged suctioning is being performed. Mouth suction can be applied directly to the oral-tracheal tube and may be most efficacious in removing thick meconium. (The person suctioning should always wear a mask.) Repeated suctioning can also be performed by passing a DeLee suction catheter either directly into the trachea (difficult to do because of the flexibility of the catheter tubing) or indirectly through a 3.5 or 4.0 mm internal diameter oral-tracheal tube. Suction is applied by the mouth on the other end of the suction apparatus.

CLINICAL CHARACTERISTICS

1. Meconium aspiration is a disease of full term and especially postmature infants. It is rare in infants born before 36 weeks' gestation.
2. Signs of respiratory distress are nonspecific and include tachypnea, nasal flaring, and retractions. The chest may appear hyperexpanded. The infant's color is often cyanotic, but not ashen or gray.

3. Radiographic examination demonstrates hyperexpanded, lucent-appearing areas interspersed with atelectatic areas throughout all the lobes.
4. The infant's skin and nail beds are usually meconium-stained. This finding is helpful, but it is not diagnostic of MAS in a term infant with respiratory distress. For example, when congenital pneumonia is present, the meconium staining will reflect a difficult fetal-to-neonatal transition but not necessarily aspiration of meconium.
5. There are no specific laboratory data useful in diagnosis. Blood gas tensions reflect increased venous admixture and a need for oxygen therapy and (using the same criteria as for HMD) ventilatory support.
6. The natural history of meconium aspiration syndrome is measured in days of respiratory distress.

THERAPY

1. Rapid correction of asphyxia is indicated. Care is supportive once the aspiration has occurred. Meconium rapidly moves down the airways to the lung periphery, and it is not easily suctioned or removed by mechanical means once it has migrated. There appears to be little usefulness in providing airway suctioning on more than a routine basis for these infants.
2. Infants with respiratory failure require mechanical ventilation. However, they often need both sedatives (morphine 0.1 mg/kg q 4 hr) and paralysis (pancuronium bromide 0.05–0.1 mg/kg prn) to achieve satisfactory ventilatory control. These medications may need to be continued for several days. It is possible, although there is no evidence, that paralyzing a vigorous term infant and controlling ventilation may limit the risk of developing air leak complications.
3. An extremely high risk of air leak exists in this disease and must always be considered in the event of rapid deterioration.
4. Positive end-expiratory pressure (PEEP) at levels of 4–6 cm H_2O may improve gas exchange in MAS in infants with respiratory failure.
5. Infants suffering from MAS often develop hypoglycemia, which further complicates management.
6. Although meconium itself is usually sterile, it supports bacterial growth in vitro, and secondary bacterial infection remains a constant risk. However, there is no evidence that routine antibiotic administration alters the course of MAS.
7. There is no evidence that chest physiotherapy or corticosteroids alter the natural history of disease.

ADDITIONAL COMMENTS

1. Meconium staining is common (10% of all deliveries at term). Severe meconium aspiration syndrome is much less common.
2. Because meconium aspiration pneumonia often occurs with little advance warning (sometimes it is not suspected until membranes are ruptured just prior to delivery), and because it occurs in term or postterm infants, it is a problem that must be anticipated and coped with in every hospital or nonhospital setting in which babies are delivered.
3. Because infants with MAS are likely to be undergrown and postmature, they have a higher risk for polycythemia (see Chapter 16) and hypoglycemia (see Chapter 13).

REFERENCES

1. Bancalari E, Berlin JA: Meconium aspiration and other asphyxial disorders. Clin Perinatology 5:317, 1978.
2. Carson B, Losey R, Bowes W: Combined obstetric and pediatric approach to prevent meconium aspiration syndrome. Am J Obstet Gynecol 126:712, 1976.
3. Yeh T, Srinivasan G, Harris V, Pildes R: Hydrocortisone therapy in meconium aspiration syndrome: A controlled study. J Pediatr 90:140, 1977.

NEONATAL PNEUMONIA

GENERAL CONSIDERATIONS

1. The lung is a common target organ for infection, perhaps because of the ease of aspirating the infected secretions that are often present in the birth canal. Newborns also have an immature local defense system—airway secretory IgA is diminished, and the chemotactic properties of neutrophils and alveolar macrophages are generally deficient.
2. Risk of any infection is highest in premature infants and may be accentuated by hypoxic depression of cellular immune systems in a setting of perinatal asphyxia.
3. Etiologic agents are many and include both gram-negative and gram-positive organisms.
4. The structure of the lung predisposes the newborn to more serious consequences. There is a relative lack of collateral ventilation, an increased mucous gland density in airways, narrower airways producing increased resistance to airflow, and diminished pulmonary reserves reflected in a lower resting arterial PO_2.

PRESENTATION

1. The degree of clinical respiratory distress is often disproportional to radiographic findings. Therefore, in any infant suspected of sepsis, a chest radiograph is warranted to detect the presence of pneumonia.
2. The clinical signs of pneumonia are indistinguishable from those of sepsis, since both illnesses often occur together. They include tachypnea (more than 60 beats/min), labored breathing with retractions, cyanosis, and apnea. It is rare for a newborn to demonstrate cough or mucous production in association with pneumonia.
3. Blood gas tensions should reflect hypoxemia and, if pneumonia is severe, hypercarbia.

ETIOLOGIC AGENTS

Table 9–5. ETIOLOGIC AGENTS OF NEONATAL PNEUMONIA

BACTERIAL
Group B streptococci
Escherichia coli
Other gram-negative organisms (especially in premature infants requiring mechanical ventilation)
Hemophilus influenza (often with associated pleural fluid)
Streptococcus pneumoniae
Listeria monocytogenes
VIRAL
Cytomegalovirus (CMV)
Respiratory syncytial virus (RSV)
Enterovirus
Herpesvirus
OTHER
Treponema pallidum (congenital syphilis)
Pneumocystis in chronically debilitated infants (this agent has not been reported as a cause of congenital pneumonia)
Chlamydia trachomatis (occurs usually beyond the first 3 weeks of life)
Aspiration pneumonia associated with gastric reflux

DIAGNOSIS

1. There can be a variable radiographic appearance: unilateral or bilateral alveolar infiltrates or a more diffuse interstitial pattern may be present. The exact pattern is not usually helpful in the differential diagnosis, except among older infants with staphylococcal pneumonia, in whom pneumatoceles will often be present.

2. Many bacterial pneumonias will be accompanied by positive blood cultures. Staphylococcal pneumonia is usually an exception.
3. Neutrophil counts can be variable. Very high or low counts (fewer than 2000 or more than 20,000 cells/mL) are suggestive of pneumonia and sepsis.
4. Tracheal aspirate examinations and cultures may prove to be useful for ill newborns, but often the culture results of this material do not correlate with disease.

THERAPY

1. Same as for sepsis; see Chapter 14.
2. Maintain adequate temperature and fluid support.
3. Administer appropriate antibiotics. Most causes of pneumonia are bacterial, and broad-spectrum antibiotics, usually ampicillin and gentamicin, are appropriate starting therapy until culture results and sensitivity testing can guide further treatment.
4. Postural drainage usually is of little help in neonates, but it is often utilized anyway.
5. Early onset pneumonias often are accompanied by overwhelming shock. Antibiotic therapy and coagulation factor replacement to treat concomitant disseminated intravascular coagulation (DIC) (see Chapter 16) seem to make little difference to the clinical course of these unfortunate infants. Newer forms of therapy, including granulocyte transfusions and specific immune globulin transfusions, may offer more hope of slowing or stopping the often inexorable downward clinical course.

ADDITIONAL COMMENTS

1. Infants who are intubated with a nasotracheal tube for more than 2 weeks are at increased risk for otitis media, which may predispose to recurrent infections.
2. Consideration must be given to noninfectious causes of pneumonia in children with chronic (more than 2 weeks) infiltrates on a chest radiograph. These causes include lymphangiectasis, desquamative interstitial pneumonia, recurrent pulmonary hemorrhage, cystic fibrosis, and recurrent aspiration pneumonia.
3. Severe undiagnosed pneumonia may require an open lung biopsy to make the diagnosis. Although this may add to the short term morbidity, it can shorten the overall course of the illness by indicating appropriate changes in therapy.
4. Prevention of streptococcal pneumonia with penicillin administered at birth only appears to trade one set of virulent organ-

isms for another, without decreasing the overall risk of infectious disease in newborns.

REFERENCES

1. Santos J, Shigeoka A, Rote N, Hill H: Protective efficacy of a modified immune serum globulin in experimental group B streptococcal infection. J Pediatr 99:873, 1981.
2. Siegal J, McCracken G, Threlkeld N, Mulvenn B, Rosenfeld C: Single dose penicillin prophylaxis against neonatal group B streptococcal infections. N Engl J Med 303:769, 1980.
3. Vollman J, Smith W, Ballard E, Light I: Early onset group B streptococcal disease: Clinical, roentgenographic, and pathologic features. J Pediatr 89:199, 1976.

PULMONARY AIR LEAK

DEFINITION

Pulmonary air leak describes several conditions that may occur spontaneously or, more commonly, in conjunction with assisted ventilation in newborns with any cause of respiratory distress.

1. Air leak occurs when the alveolar walls rupture and gas moves along perivascular and lymphatic sheaths until it reaches the pleural space.
2. The most commonly recognized conditions include pneumomediastinum (PMN, air collection in the anterior mediastinum); pneumothorax (PT, right-sided, left-sided, or bilateral, in which air is trapped between parietal and visceral pleura); pneumopericardium (PPC, air between heart and pericardial sac); pneumoperitoneum (PPT, air that tracks into the peritoneal space by way of the posterior mediastinal openings in the diaphragm); and pulmonary interstitial emphysema (PIE, a localized pulmonary form of air leak in which small pockets of presumably extra-alveolar gas remain localized and scattered in pulmonary tissue). PIE may occur diffusely or be localized in one lobe only.

PRESENTATION

1. Air leaks produce variable effects on clinical status ranging from none (often with PMN) to immediately life-threatening (bilateral PT, PPC, PPT).
2. Air leaks usually produce hypoxemia but occasionally may only increase the arterial carbon dioxide tension ($PaCO_2$).
3. There may be a transient elevation in systemic blood pressure

with a PT. Recent observations suggest a relationship between blood pressure changes with PT and the development of intracranial hemorrhage, although this relationship is not firmly established.

DIAGNOSIS

1. Diagnosis is readily made by chest radiography. It is useful to have both an anterior-posterior and a lateral view so that the exact location and extent of the air collection can be determined.
2. Transillumination of the chest wall will reveal a translucent glow if an anterior PT is present. This technique may save time if a large PT has occurred. However, a normal transillumination does not always rule out a small but still clinically important PT.
3. Traditional signs of air leak in adults are often unhelpful in newborns because the sick lung may fail to collapse completely and shift the mediastinum toward the ipsilateral side, and because breath sounds emanating from only one lung are audible by auscultation in both lung fields. Therefore, the absence of unequal breath sounds does not rule out the presence of an air leak.
4. The presentation of PPC is immediate, with hypotension and muffled and distant heart sounds. There is often no time for a chest radiograph. Immediate evacuation of the air is life-saving (see the following section).

THERAPY

1. Symptomatic PT or PT occurring with extensive parenchymal disease requires evacuation of air and re-expansion of the lung. Usually this is accomplished by placement of a flexible plastic thoracostomy tube of appropriate size (10 or 12 Fr in a term infant) in the anterior axillary line, away from the nipple, and with the tip of the tube placed in the anterior superior location. Local anesthetic is infiltrated into the skin, followed by a small (1 cm) skin incision. Then the tube with a rigid trocar inside is inserted just over the top of the 4th rib into the pleural space. It is helpful to puncture the pleura with a hemostat and then use that instrument to guide the tube tip inward through the pleural rent. This can be done without the trocar in place. Suture the tube in place with a pursestring suture. Be careful that the tube is not pulled out during the procedure.
2. If the infant has acutely deteriorated, it may be necessary to remove air by needle aspiration before placing the thoracostomy tube. This can be done using a butterfly needle (Nos. 21

or 23 gauge) attached to flexible tubing, with a clamp placed just behind the needle to prevent inappropriately deep needle insertion (Figs. 9–1 and 9–2). The end of the flexible tubing should be placed under sterile water to prevent drawing more air into the pleural space.

3. PMN only rarely requires evacuation even when air dissects into neck.
4. PPC requires immediate evacuation using a substernal approach applying negative pressure on the barrel of a 20 cc syringe attached to a No. 22 gauge Teflon catheter with needle. Direct the needle tip toward the middle of the left clavicle until air enters the syringe. The needle can then be withdrawn, and the flexible catheter can be sutured in to evacuate any recurrent leaks.

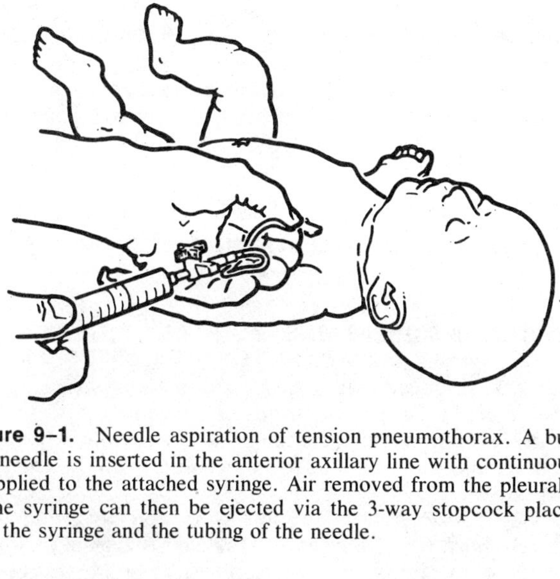

Figure 9–1. Needle aspiration of tension pneumothorax. A butterfly metal needle is inserted in the anterior axillary line with continuous suction applied to the attached syringe. Air removed from the pleural space into the syringe can then be ejected via the 3-way stopcock placed between the syringe and the tubing of the needle.

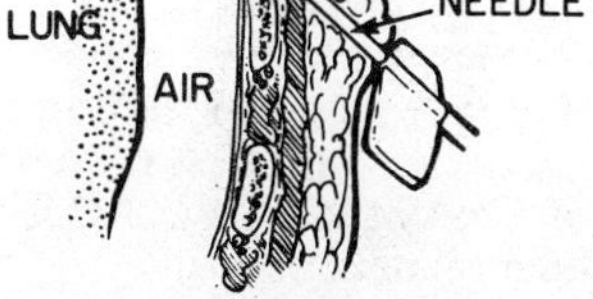

Figure 9–2. Schematic illustration of proper needle angle and placement for withdrawal of free air from the pleural space. Note that the needle passes just over the top of a rib, avoiding the intercostal vessels that run just below the rib.

5. PPT is more problematic. The physician must know if the air is from a ruptured abdominal viscus or is a pulmonary complication. The latter does not necessarily require operative intervention. Free abdominal air in sick newborns most commonly occurs with necrotizing enterocolitis (see Chapter 12); the abdominal radiograph may reveal evidence of NEC. A diagnostic tap of the abdominal space to detect the presence of free abdominal fluid may help determine the need for surgery. *Note:* If such a patient must be transported, either by air or over mountain passes, it is critically important to evacuate all the free peritoneal air. The inevitable expansion of this trapped gas with lowered ambient pressure will worsen the respiratory status.

ADDITIONAL COMMENTS

Pulmonary air leaks are very common problems in sick newborns. Pneumothorax in particular is not limited to the intensive care setting. Any hospital caring for infants with even minimal respiratory distress must be prepared to deal immediately with this complication.

CONGENITAL MALFORMATIONS OF THE AIRWAYS

GENERAL CONSIDERATIONS

1. Each type of congenital airway malformation is rare by itself, but as a group the various forms of congenital airway malformations are sufficiently common—and treatable when recognized in time—to be included in any discussion of emergency conditions.
2. Any of the lesions described in this section can occur in prematurely born or term infants. Tracheoesophageal fistula may predispose to prematurity, as many cases of TE fistula are in preterm infants.
3. Airway lesions are often associated with other malformations. The task of the physician is to diagnose the anatomic site of the defect, stabilize the infant by providing fluids and warmth, maintain a patent airway to the extent possible, and ascertain the presence of other severe life-threatening deficits.
4. Multiple defects at different levels of the airway (e.g., choanal atresia and tracheoesophageal fistula) may occur in the same patient.
5. Infants with the lesions described in this chapter typically develop signs of respiratory distress immediately at birth.

INDIVIDUAL LESIONS OF IMPORTANCE

1. *Choanal atresia* is a narrowing or blockage by protrusion of bone or membrane into nasal air passages. Cyanosis and gasping efforts occur immediately upon birth when the condition is bilateral; intermittent signs of distress result when it is unilateral. Distress occurs because the infant is normally an obligate nose-breather. Diagnosis is made by failure to pass a catheter through either nasal passage into the posterior oropharynx. Treatment consists of placing the infant in a prone position and inserting and taping securely in place a large oral airway. If this proves difficult because of associated facial undergrowth, an oral-tracheal tube can be placed and secured. Surgical treatment consists of perforation of the obstruction and introduction of obturators, followed by serial dilation.
2. *Micrognathia* (mandibular undergrowth as may occur with the Pierre-Robin syndrome) or a *large tongue* (as in infants with congenital hypothyroidism) may cause respiratory impairment by blocking the upper airway. The conditions may be suspected when airway distress is relieved by prone positioning, with the head down. Placement of an oral airway or oral-tracheal tube provides a patent airway. Humidified gas should be directed to the intratracheal tube to help prevent drying of secretions, and special attention is always needed for suctioning, as excessive secretions may occlude the airway.
3. *Tracheoesophageal fistula* can take several forms, but the distal fistula coupled with proximal esophageal atresia is the only commonly occurring type. This condition is recognized in the first minutes or hours after birth by a constant frothing of unswallowable sputum and secretions, by intermittent signs of respiratory distress (including cyanosis), and finally by an inability to place a nasal or oral catheter into the stomach. Occasionally infants remain undiagnosed until the first feeding, which will produce immediate choking and gasping. Confirmation of the diagnosis is made by obtaining an anterior-posterior and lateral chest radiograph with a radiopaque catheter advanced as far as possible into the esophagus. (Check the back of the throat to be sure that the catheter is not coiled there, but do not apply excessive pressure to the catheter, which could cause possible perforation.) Gas in the stomach and intestine confirms the presence of the distal fistula.

   Immediate management consists of maintaining the infant in an upright position, with a large catheter suctioning drainage in the proximal esophageal pouch to prevent overflow and aspiration of secretions. When the infant is stable, ligation of the fistula is carried out, and, occasionally, a gastrostomy tube is placed to prevent aspiration. The possibility of attempting direct anastomosis of the two ends of the esophagus requires careful judgment on the part of the surgeon and depends on the size of the patient and the gap between the two ends of the esophagus. The operation can have several complications: the two ends of the esophagus may be stretched too tightly, producing suture line leakage and secondary inflammation, and the mediastinum can be scarred. In most infants, the lung parenchyma is normal if aspiration pneumonia has not occurred.

4. *Diaphragmatic hernia* occurs because of a defect in the development of the diaphragm involving failure of the pleuroperitoneal canal to close. The herniation is usually on the left side through the foramen of Bochdalek, and abdominal contents enter the thoracic cavity during fetal life. This results in at least unilateral pulmonary hypoplasia and immediate respiratory distress *at birth* (cyanotic appearance and gasping respirations), usually coupled with a flat or scaphoid abdomen. Emergency care consists of recognizing the possibility of a diaphragmatic hernia, and immediately placing an oral or nasal tracheal tube for assisted ventilation and a gastric tube to maintain decompression of the misplaced bowel. Inflation of the thoracic bowel with air produces further pulmonary compromise. Adequate oxygenation is difficult, but high inspiratory or expiratory airway pressures often produce pneumothorax and further deterioration. Most children requiring surgery in the first 24–48 hrs of life do not survive, but their mortality is increased without surgery. The immediate postoperative course is sometimes characterized by a "honeymoon" period before intractable hypoxemia recurs. Pulmonary hypertension often occurs postoperatively, and its management is controversial and usually unsuccessful. One untested possibility is unilateral pneumonectomy. No satisfactory approach to this difficult situation has yet been devised.
5. *Renal agenesis, renal dysgenesis,* and *blockage of the urinary outlet by urethral valves* are often associated with pulmonary hypoplasia. These conditions are suspected when oligohydramnios occurs because of less than normal fetal urine contribution to amniotic fluid, and when physical examination reveals an undergrown infant with a small, pinched face and low-set ears. These infants develop severe respiratory distress; a chest radiograph will demonstrate small chest space, ribs close together, and unexpanded lungs. This condition is not treatable, and severely affected infants die within hours or days of pulmonary insufficiency. Lung weight may be only half that expected based on body weight.
6. A variety of *intrinsic pulmonary overdistention problems,* especially *congenital lobar emphysema* (localized overdistention of one lobe perhaps secondary to a defect in cartilaginous bronchial rings) may produce acute respiratory embarrassment beginning within hours of birth. Diagnosis is by chest radiograph; care is needed to distinguish between unilateral atelectasis with secondary hyperexpansion of the contralateral lung

versus unilateral emphysema. Treatment is surgical resection. Initial stabilization in critically ill infants may consist of unilateral ventilation by selective intubation of the unaffected lung, if it proves impossible to maintain gas exchange any other way.

7. *Tracheomalacia,* characterized by stridulous inspiration, occurs for unknown reasons, perhaps related to tracheal cartilaginous deficiency. Usually, no immediate treatment is necessary. The physician must, however, distinguish this condition from others, including extrinsic or intrinsic compression of the trachea caused by mediastinal masses. Ruling out these latter lesions may require laryngoscopy or bronchoscopy.
8. A rare cause of acute respiratory embarrassment in the newborn period is unilateral or bilateral paresis or paralysis of the diaphragm. Diagnosis is by fluoroscopy; treatment is usually surgical with plication of the diaphragm, although some infants may benefit from application of continuous pressure without intermittent mechanical ventilation. This condition may occur following particularly severe birth injury (see Chapter 3).

ADDITIONAL COMMENTS

All of these conditions are usually unsuspected prior to delivery. They produce immediate and in some cases life-threatening distress. They are treatable and in most cases curable. Therefore, any physician or nurse administering to newborns—in any setting—must be prepared to encounter one or another of these conditions and must know the correct steps in managing them.

REFERENCES

1. Burtain W, Isaacs H, Payne V, Lindesmith G, Rosenkrantz J: Lobar emphysema, cystic adenomatoid malformation, pulmonary sequestration, and bronchogenic cyst in infancy and childhood: A clinical group. J Pediatr Surg 9:85, 1974.
2. Hicks L, Mansfield PB: Esophageal atresia and tracheoesophageal fistula. Review of thirteen years' experience. J Thorac Cardiovasc Surg 81:358, 1981.
3. Stahlman, M: Respiratory Disorders in the Newborn. *In* Kendig EL Jr, Chernick V (eds): Disorders of the Respiratory Tract in Children, 3rd ed. Philadelphia, Saunders, 1977.

10

APNEA

GENERAL CONSIDERATIONS

1. Apnea is a pause in breathing that may be accompanied by changes in skin color, arterial oxygenation, heart rate, and blood pressure. Apnea may be central in origin, in which case failure to initiate the next respiration is reflected in absent chest movement. Obstructive apnea may occur with mechanical blockage at any level of the respiratory tract. Usually there is no difficulty in differentiating apnea from periodic breathing; the latter is unaccompanied by physiologic changes and persists for less than 20 sec.
2. Apnea is a symptom that requires elucidation of the cause as well as monitoring and treatment of the condition itself. Most apnea in premature infants is idiopathic.
3. The likelihood of idiopathic apnea developing in an infant is inversely correlated with gestational age. It is rare in infants of more than 37 weeks' gestation. Infants of 28–30 weeks' gestation will routinely have detectable apnea during the first days of life.
4. Because physicians cannot specify a "safe" point beyond which serious apneic episodes are unlikely to occur, nurses have to expend a great deal of time monitoring this condition.

PATIENT PRESENTATION

1. Apnea may be associated with any of several common conditions in neonates, including hypoxemia, hypoglycemia, sepsis, seizures, intracranial hemorrhage, and electrolyte imbalance. The causal relationships between these abnormalities and apneic episodes are uncertain.
2. Idiopathic apnea often begins after the first 24 hr of life and has a variable time of peak severity, but typically this peak occurs during the first week of life.
3. Bradycardia may occur only after a long (60 sec) pause after the end of the last breath, or it may develop almost spontaneously with the initiation of the pause in breathing. Although these two different patterns may have different physiologic meanings, research has not yet clearly differentiated the cause(s) of these patterns.

DIAGNOSIS

Apnea can be diagnosed by observation of absent respiratory movements. Because of the unpredictable pattern of apnea, electronic monitoring of respiratory activity (most commonly chest movement) and heart rate monitoring are used for diagnosis. Machines are prone to failure; constant vigilance is required to assure that monitor alarms are properly working and are set in a "ready" mode. Even the most sophisticated equipment requires human monitoring.

Air flow monitoring at the nose using thermistors is useful in differentiating obstructive from central apnea.

RISKS OF UNINTERRUPTED APNEA

1. Hypoxemia and hypoxic brain damage.
2. Further respiratory depression and increased difficulty in terminating the episode.
3. Aspiration of stomach contents and pneumonia.
4. Altered distribution of cardiac output, perhaps leading to ischemic damage in some organs.
5. Death.

THERAPY

1. Assume apnea is secondary to another cause, and treat any treatable associated conditions. This principle applies especially in near term or term infants in whom there is a great likelihood of detecting a serious associated condition. A minimal evaluation should include culturing and treating for possible sepsis and measuring serum electrolyte and glucose levels.
2. Considerable skill and experience is required of medical and nursing personnel in distinguishing infants who will spontaneously resume respiratory activity in a few seconds without other significant changes from those who will require some form of stimulation.
3. Many episodes of apnea are terminated simply by tactile stimulation of the infant, specifically by sitting him up and stroking his back, face, chest, chin, and extremities. Gentle pinching of the feet may help.
4. Should generalized cyanosis intensify, or bradycardia of less than 100 beats/min persist or worsen during the next 30–60 sec, in spite of increasingly active handling or stroking and the use of free-flowing oxygen to the face, then (1) promptly empty the infant's stomach of any retained feedings, and (2) begin artificial ventilation with bag and mask. The inspired oxygen should be similar to that which the infant was breathing before

the episode unless cyanosis persists, in which case the inspired oxygen concentration should be increased.

If attacks occur so frequently (several per hour) or with such severity that regular feeding schedules become impossible to meet, one or both of two more aggressive approaches are indicated:

a. Pharmacologic manipulation of the infant's respiratory control center with methylxanthine (theophylline, aminophylline, or caffeine) therapy administered either orally or intravenously. (See Table 10–1 for dosages.)

Table 10–1. PHARMACOLOGIC MANAGEMENT OF APNEA

DRUG*	ROUTE	DOSAGE	THERAPEUTIC LEVEL
Aminophylline	IV	5 mg/kg loading dose then 1–2 mg/kg q 8–12 hr	6–12 mcg/mL
Theophylline	oral	same as aminophylline	6–12 mcg/mL
Caffeine	oral	10–15 mg/kg loading dose, then 5–10 mg/kg q 12 hr	8–15 mcg/mL

*The half-lives of these drugs in premature infants are highly variable (values of 24–60 hr have been reported) and depend on gestational and postnatal age. Possible side effects include tachycardia, jitteriness, convulsions, and feeding intolerance.

b. Treatment with assisted ventilation, usually at a low rate of 5–12 breaths/min, utilizing a minimal peak inspiratory pressure of 15–18 cm H_2O and low gas flow rates.

The long term evaluation of infants treated with methylxanthines has not shown an excess of neurologic problems, although animal studies using massive dosages of these agents have shown adverse neurologic effects.

Other approaches to the control of idiopathic apnea have been advocated, including supplementation of inspired oxygen concentration to maintain arterial PO_2 at greater than physiologic levels and lowering of the ambient temperature of the incubator. However, these schemes are associated with significant risks of their own (e.g., retrolental fibroplasia in premature infants and chilling of the infant with increased caloric expenditure). We do not recommend them. The use of oscillating waterbeds has been advocated by some, but there is little evidence that such an approach is effective.

ADDITIONAL COMMENTS

1. The cause of central apnea in prematures is unknown. Many potential contributing factors have not been thoroughly studied. These include the relative importance of chest wall afferent neuromuscular signals and chest wall (and lung resting vol-

ume) stability; diaphragmatic fatigue; the role of the immature paradoxical ventilatory response of the neonate to hypoxia, consisting of initial hyperventilation followed in a few minutes by a return to the previous (or lower) level of minute ventilation; and altered levels of local neurotransmitters in the brain stem region of the central nervous system.

2. Obstructive apnea is a major concern in infants with upper airway anomalies such as micrognathia (Pierre Robin syndrome) or a large tongue (congenital hypothyroidism). These problems must be managed by placement of an oral airway or prone positioning of the infant.
3. Persistent, severe apnea beyond the first weeks of life in any infant, preterm or term, should suggest a more complex pathology. An evaluation to determine the cause or relevant associated conditions might include determining the possibility of seizure activity presenting clinically as apnea (EEG); gastric reflux with out without aspiration (a variety of studies can be used to detect this, the most useful being 24 hr esophageal pH monitoring); and special imaging studies to evaluate for CNS malformations or hemorrhage.
4. Present evidence suggests no strong correlation between the degree or severity of apnea in prematurity and the risk of sudden infant death syndrome (SIDS) during the first year of life, although this relationship has not been thoroughly studied. Premature infants have an increased risk of SIDS, but the great majority of infants dying of SIDS are not premature and have no problems in the newborn period.
5. It is not known why apnea is not as severe in the first hours of life as later in the first week of life.

REFERENCES

1. Bory C, Baltassat P, Porthault M, Bethenod M, Frederich A, Aranda J: Metabolism of theophylline to caffeine in premature infants. J Pediatr 94:988, 1979.
2. Gerhardt T, McCarthy J, Bancalari E: Effect of aminophylline on respiratory center activity and metabolic rate in premature infants with idiopathic apnea. Pediatrics 63:537, 1979.
3. Kattwinkel J: Neonatal apnea: Pathogenesis and therapy. J Pediatr 90:342, 1977.
4. Myers T, Milsap R, Krauss A, Auld P, Reidenberg M: Low dose theophylline therapy in idiopathic apnea of prematurity. J Pediatr 96:99, 1980.

11

CARDIOVASCULAR DISORDERS

CONGENITAL HEART DISEASE OVERVIEW

GENERAL CONSIDERATIONS

1. Incidence is 7.5/1000 live births or 1/140 births.
2. Congenital heart disease (CHD) includes a number of anatomically distinct entities and variations of specific malformations.
3. With early recognition and advances in surgical methods, survival rates continue to improve.
4. CHD is often associated with other congenital defects.
5. CHD is generally classified as cyanotic or acyanotic, with further categorization by quantitative differences in pulmonary blood flow.
6. Patent ductus arteriosus is given special consideration owing to its frequency and postnatal acquisition.
7. *Etiology:*
   a. Largely unknown.
   b. Chromosomal abnormalities (Down's, trisomy 13–15, trisomy 16–18, Turner's).
   c. Hereditary: congenital hypertrophic subaortic stenosis, familial cardiomyopathy, Kartagener's syndrome, glycogen storage disease, supravalvular aortic stenosis and hypercalcemia, Turner's syndrome, Noonan's syndrome, and rhabdomyoma associated with tuberous sclerosis; also Apert's, Holt-Oram, Seckel's, Treacher Collins, Smith-Lemli-Opitz, Hunter-Hurler syndromes and osteogenesis imperfecta.
   d. Maternal drug use: thalidomide, alcohol, steroids, quinine, teratogens, antimetabolites, phenytoin, trimethadione, lithium, warfarin, progesterone-estrogen, and dextroamphetamines.
   e. Infection: rubella, possibly mumps, influenza, and Coxsackie B virus.

PRESENTATION

Order of frequency of malformations in the neonatal period:

1. PDA.
2. Transposition of great vessels.
3. Ventricular septal defect (VSD).
4. Complex heart disease.
5. Hypoplastic left heart syndrome.
6. Coarctation of aorta.

7. Tetralogy of Fallot.
8. Hypoplastic right heart.
9. Pulmonary stenosis.
10. Endocardial cushion defect.
11. Primary myocardial disease.
12. Total anomalous pulmonary venous return.
13. Truncus arteriosus.
14. Aortic stenosis.
15. Pulmonary artery stenosis.
16. Ebstein's anomaly.
17. Arteriovenous (A-V) fistula.

Incidence is approximately 3 times greater in premature infants. However, infants with transposition of great vessels are almost always term and heavy.

Subtle onset of signs is common: e.g., poor feeding, poor weight gain, and tachypnea.

Congenital heart disease is always suspect when other congenital anomalies are present.

DIAGNOSIS

1. History.
2. There is a wide range of clinical signs, but the most characteristic are rapid, unlabored, shallow breathing unaccompanied by grunting, flaring of nostrils, or retracting; and gray, ashen, or cyanotic skin.
3. Heart murmurs typically are present but may be absent if left- and right-sided pressures are equal shortly after birth.
4. Chest radiograph to determine cardiac contour and size and the degree of pulmonary vascularity.
5. Electrocardiogram.
6. Echocardiograph, including two-dimensional and Doppler.
7. Heart catheterization:
   a. If echocardiography is uncertain.
   b. If heart failure is present.
   c. If a surgically correctable lesion is suspected (e.g., transposition of the great vessels).

MANAGEMENT

1. Observation and serial evaluation.
2. Digitalis and diuretic.
3. Prostaglandin E to maintain patency of ductus arteriosus when a ductal shunt is critical to survival.
4. Atrial balloon septostomy if transposition is present.
5. Palliative surgery.
6. Corrective surgery.

7. Some conditions are not amenable to medical or surgical treatment, e.g., hypoplastic left-sided heart syndrome.

DISTURBANCES OF RATE OR RHYTHM

The only common abnormality in the neonatal period is paroxysmal atrial tachycardia, often more appropriately called supraventricular tachycardia.

Etiology

1. Usually unknown.
2. May be accompanied by Wolff-Parkinson-White syndrome of aberrant A-V conduction.

Presentation

1. Onset of tachypnea.
2. Progressive signs of congestive heart failure (CHF), occasionally cyanosis.

Diagnosis. Cardiac rate should be >220/min and often is close to 300/min. Condition must persist during periods of quiet to confirm diagnosis.

Treatment

1. Oxygen and treatment for signs of CHF if tachycardia persists.
2. Digitalization.
3. Countershock is occasionally indicated.

Congenital Heartblock

This uncommon lesion presents as bradycardia, unresponsive to crying or stimulation. A diligent search needs to be made for complex congenital structural heart disease, with which it is commonly associated. No treatment is required if no symptoms appear and the rate is ≥70/min. Isoproterenol or a pacemaker may be necessary for symptomatic heart block.

REFERENCES

1. Anon: Editorial: Congenital heart-disease: incidence and aetiology. Lancet 2:692, 1975.
2. Morgan BC: Incidence, etiology, and classification of congenital heart disease. Pediatr Clin North Am 25:721, 1978.
3. Rowland TW: The pediatrician and congenital heart disease—1972. Pediatrics 64:180, 1979.
4. Rudolph A: Congenital Diseases of the Heart. Chicago, Year Book, 1974.
5. Shannon DC, Lusser M, Goldblatt A, Burnell JB: The cyanotic infant—heart disease or lung disease. N Eng J Med 287:951, 1972.

CYANOTIC HEART DISEASE

GENERAL CONSIDERATIONS

1. Many types of heart disease may make the infant appear cyanotic because of poor cardiac output (hypoplastic left-sided heart syndrome) or because of variable pulmonary blood flow (some ductal dependent lesions, severe pulmonic stenosis, some forms of truncus arteriosus). Therefore, simple straightforward listing of acyanotic and cyanotic lesions can sometimes be misleading.
2. An important differential in the cyanotic newborn is persistent fetal circulation, which presents with cyanosis and diminished pulmonary blood flow but with a structurally normal heart.
3. The relationship between cyanosis and arterial PO_2 is not fixed. The clinical finding of cyanosis depends on an absolute level of unsaturated hemoglobin ($\geq$ 5 g/100 mL). Depending on the quantity of hemoglobin and the hemoglobin-oxygen affinity, the PaO_2 at which cyanosis occurs can vary.
4. The most important task for the physician is to recognize the possibility of cyanotic heart disease (altered blood flow to lungs detected by chest radiograph, change in heart size, murmur, cyanosis unrelieved by oxygen) and arrange for immediate consultation.
5. Echocardiography is a useful tool in diagnosing or excluding many forms of cyanotic congenital heart disease. In most cases, the deranged anatomy can be seen with two-dimensional echocardiography.
6. In lesions with decreased pulmonary blood flow, a continuous infusion of prostaglandin E_1 may help maintain patency of the ductus arteriosus and diminish pulmonary vascular resistance, allowing the infant to maintain some mixing of blood until more definitive procedures can be performed.

CLASSIFICATION OF COMMON LESIONS PRODUCING CYANOSIS

1. Pulmonary vascularity increased:
   a. Transposition of the great vessels (right ventricular hypertrophy).
   b. Truncus arteriosus, some forms (right ventricular hypertrophy).
   c. Subdiaphragmatic total anomalous pulmonary venous return (right ventricular hypertrophy).
2. Pulmonary vascularity decreased:
   a. Tetralogy of Fallot (right ventricular hypertrophy).

b. Tricuspid atresia (left ventricular hypertrophy).
c. Ebstein's anomaly (right ventricular hypertrophy).

SELECTED LESIONS

Transposition of Great Vessels

General Comments

1. Most common cyanotic lesion.
2. Typically presents in large plethoric-appearing infants.
3. May be rapid deterioration in 2–3 days without palliation.

Anatomy. The aorta arises anteriorly from the right ventricle and carries deoxygenated blood to the systemic circulation; the posterior-arising pulmonary artery carries oxygenated blood back to the lungs from the left ventricle. The extent of communication between the two circulations at a coexisting ventricular septal defect (VSD), atrial septal defect (ASD), or patent ductus arteriosus (PDA) determines the degree of cyanosis and symptoms and the length of survival without treatment.

Presentation

1. Early and profound cyanosis.
2. Rapid onset of congestive failure.
3. Systolic murmur usually heard.
4. Cardiomegaly on chest radiograph.

Immediate treatment is balloon atrial septostomy to improve mixing and decrease cyanosis.

Total Anomalous Pulmonary Venous Return

General Considerations

Definitions. Pulmonary veins connect to systemic venous system via:

1. Right atrium.
2. Right superior vena cava or azygous vein.
3. Left superior vena cava or coronary sinus.
4. Portal vein or ductus venosus.

Incidence. One in 7000 births. Accounts for 1–5% of congenital cardiac defects. Incidence for males equals that for females.

Hemodynamics. Oxygenated pulmonary venous blood mixes with desaturated blood in the right atrium. If there is an obstruction to systemic venous flow (as in the infradiaphragmatic type), pulmonary venous congestion develops. Pulmonary hypertension results, and patent ductus arteriosus may be present. The degree of oxygenation depends on the shunting of blood through the foramen ovale to the left atrium, as well as on the amount of pulmonary blood flow.

Presentation. The time of onset of signs varies according to the degree of venous obstruction and atrial shunt. Signs often are delayed a few days after birth and consist of tachypnea progressing to cyanosis. The infradiaphragmatic type presents with more severe signs and more obvious cyanosis at an earlier age. If pulmonary blood flow is excessive, cyanosis does not usually develop. Heart failure may develop during the first three weeks of life. Murmurs are variable or absent, and the liver is enlarged. Blood pressure and peripheral pulses are usually normal. Pulmonic second sound (P_2) is accentuated; quadruple rhythms may develop.

Diagnosis

Chest Radiographs. These display two patterns:

1. Pulmonary venous congestion with normal cardiac size or slight enlargement. Caution: this can be mistaken for pneumonia or other parenchymal disease.
2. Increased pulmonary blood with moderate to marked cardiac enlargement.
3. "Snowman" or "figure-eight" pattern is not seen in neonates.

Electrocardiogram. This displays right axis deviation, right atrial overload, and sharply peaked P waves in leads V_3R and V_1 of the ECG.

Echocardiograph

1. M-mode:
   a. Large right ventricle.
   b. Large pulmonary artery.
   c. Anomalous pulmonary venous channel.
2. Two-dimensional:
   a. Anomalous venous structure.
   b. Absence of pulmonary veins emptying into left atrium.

Heart Catheterization. Used for diagnostic confirmation.

Treatment

1. Digoxin and diuretics will help nonobstructed congestive failure.
2. Surgical correction.
3. Balloon septostomy sometimes helps, but not in obstructive congestive failure.

Additional Comments. Infants with pulmonary venous obstruction have a high mortality rate within the first 2 weeks of life. Onset of failure in newborns heralds a poor prognosis, and therefore an attempt at early surgical correction is justified.

Tricuspid Atresia

Anatomy. Atresia of the pulmonary valve, underdevelopment of the right ventricle, and atrial septal defect. Defect may be associated with patent ductus arteriosus. The lesion may also occur with transposition.

Presentation

1. Severe cyanosis and diminished pulmonary blood flow.
2. Left atrial and ventricular hypertrophy on ECG.
3. Important to differentiate from persistent fetal circulation.
4. Systolic murmur usually present.

Treatment. Immediate palliative surgery to increase pulmonary blood flow and relieve cyanosis.

Tetralogy of Fallot

Anatomy. VSD, obstruction to RV outflow at or below the level of the pulmonic valve, overriding aorta, and RVH.

Presentation

1. Cyanosis may range from none to severe in the neonatal period.
2. Congestive heart failure is rare.
3. Diminished pulmonary blood flow on chest x-ray.
4. Loud systolic murmur usually present.
5. A right-sided aortic arch is present in 25% of cases.

Treatment. Symptomatic infants may require palliative surgery. Mildly affected infants can be observed until definitive surgery can be performed beyond the neonatal period.

Truncus Arteriosus

Anatomy. A single ventricle or a very large VSD is associated with a single great vessel arising from the heart. Variably sized pulmonary arterial vessels emerge from this single large vessel.

Presentation

1. The degree of cyanosis and of increased FIO_2 responsiveness depends on the amount of pulmonary blood flow.
2. Radiographic evaluation of pulmonary blood flow (PBF) can range from under- to overperfused.
3. Abrupt clinical changes may occur when pulmonary vascular resistance falls, and PBF can increase in magnitude.

Treatment. Must be individualized and will depend entirely on the degree of pulmonary flow after birth.

REFERENCES

See the list of general references following the first section of this chapter.

ACYANOTIC HEART DISEASE

CLASSIFICATION

Pulmonary Vascularity

1. Increased:
   a. Ventricular septal defect (VSD): left ventricular hypertrophy (LVH) → right ventricular hypertrophy (RVH) by ECG.
   b. Patent ductus arteriosus (PDA) (LVH).
   c. Atrioventricular canal (LVH).
   d. Partial anomalous venous return (AVR) (RVH).
   e. Atrial septal defect (ASD) (RVH).
   f. Aorticopulmonary window–combined ventricular hypertrophy (RVH and LVH).
2. Decreased:
   a. Pulmonary stenosis (RVH); if severe, may be cyanotic.
   b. Pulmonary artery coarctation and hypoplastic right heart.
3. Normal:
   a. Aortic stenosis (LVH).
   b. Aortic insufficiency (LVH).
   c. Coarctation of aorta (RVH).
   d. Hypoplastic left-sided heart syndrome (RVH); may also appear cyanotic.
   e. Congenital mitral stenosis (RVH).
   f. Primary myocardiopathy (myocarditis, endocardial fibroelastosis [EFE]) (LVH).

SELECTED DISORDERS

Ventricular Septal Defect

General Considerations

Incidence. Accounts for 10–20% of all congenital heart disease. May be an isolated defect or part of a more complex malformation. Most defects are found in the membranous portion of the septum, but the size and location of defects vary.

Hemodynamics. Variations in size determine the direction of the shunt. At first the shunt is bidirectional; then, as pulmonary vascular resistance (PVR) falls, the shunt becomes L→R, resulting in pulmonary overperfusion (edema) and left ventricular failure.

Presentation

Small Defect. A soft murmur that generally does not increase in intensity until 2–3 weeks and then becomes holosystolic and harsh over the lower left sternal border. P_2 = normal.
Moderate Defect. A murmur usually develops towards the end of the first week.
Large Defect. Tachypnea, poor feeding, pallor, poor weight gain, congestive heart failure, and possibly cyanotic episodes.

Diagnosis

Murmur. Precordial systolic murmur, usually not heard at birth, becomes pansystolic, loud, and harsh over the lower left sternal border. P_2 is dependent on pulmonary artery pressure.
Chest Radiograph. Depending on the size of the defect, the radiograph may be normal or may reveal increased vascularity with left ventricular enlargement.
Electrocardiogram. Findings depend on hemodynamics: a small defect often shows only the normal pattern of right ventricular dominance. A large defect means LVH and RVH.
Echocardiogram. M-mode: left atrium to aorta ratio normal to increased. Two-dimensional: allows visualization of the septal defect.
Differential Diagnosis. Coarctation, patent ductus arteriosus, truncus arteriosus.

Therapy

Medical. Digitalis and diuretics.
Palliative Surgery. Pulmonary artery banding.
Primary Surgical Repair. Over 6 months of age.

Pulmonic Stenosis—Isolated

General Considerations. Isolated pulmonic stenosis is a valvular or infundibular anatomic obstruction of the right ventricular outflow tract resulting in a pressure differential across the pulmonary valve. Incidence is 5% of all cases of congenital heart disease, of which 90% are valvular and 10% are subvalvular. It occurs with other complex cardiac defects, most commonly with tetralogy of Fallot.

Pure pulmonic stenosis is important to recognize early in life, since early surgery can prevent pulmonary artery dilatation.

A severe form involves fused pulmonary valve cusps.

Hemodynamics. Obstruction to the pulmonary blood flow causes right ventricular hypertrophy with narrowing of the right ventricular cavity. It may be accompanied by a patent foramen ovale with a right-to-left shunt.

Presentation. The infant may have no signs. A murmur is usually heard from birth but may be absent. The characteristic rough murmur of older children is not heard in newborn infants, who produce a soft, early systolic murmur. Cyanosis may occur with severe stenosis. Heart failure may develop after several days.

Diagnosis

1. *Chest radiograph* shows general cardiac enlargement and decreased pulmonary vascularity.
2. *Electrocardiogram* may be normal with mild stenosis, with various degrees of right ventricular hypertrophy, and with P-pulmonale in 50% of severe cases.
3. *Echocardiogram* determines the thickness of the right ventricular walls and the size of the pulmonary artery (PA).
4. *Two-dimensional echocardiogram* can detect doming of the pulmonary valve, visualize the tricuspid valves, and measure the size of the right ventricle.

Treatment

1. Treatment of associated heart failure.
2. Pulmonary valvotomy, if severe. Procedure is usually delayed 4–6 months in LBW infants. Good outcome.
3. Observation of mild or moderate forms with periodic assessment.

Hypoplastic Left Heart Syndrome

General Considerations

Definition. This is a syndrome of underdevelopment of the left side of the heart that may include left ventricle underdevelopment, aortic atresia, hypoplasia of the aortic arch, and mitral valve stenosis or atresia. It is the major cause of death from cardiac malformations in the neonatal period. It is important to differentiate from treatable lesions.

Hemodynamics. A fetal left-to-right shunt produces a large right atrium and right ventricle; postnatally, there is inadequate left ventricular output. Heart failure ensues with 1–5 days.

Presentation. The infant may be normal the first day or be in severe distress shortly after birth. Onset may be insidious, with tachypnea and severe failure not developing for 3 or 4 days. Tachycardia, occasionally with a gallop rhythm, is detected. Murmur is variable. Cyanosis often develops preterminally, usually preceded by a grayish pallor. Radial pulses may be weaker than femoral pulses. Blood pressure will be low.

Diagnosis

1. *Chest radiographs* show left- and right-sided cardiac enlargement at birth, as well as increased pulmonary vascularity.

2. *Electrocardiograms* show RVH and right axis deviation.
3. *Echocardiography* yields variable findings: large right ventricle, small left ventricle, and mitral valve distortion. Small aortic root is the main finding. If the left ventricle is very small, it is difficult to locate the ventricular septum.
4. *Heart catheterization* is used if there are doubts about a correctable lesion.

Treatment

None.

Additional Comments

The infant usually succumbs in the first week of life in spite of treatment of congestive heart failure.

Endocardial Cushion Defects Including Common Atrioventricular Canal

Anatomy. Variable with low atrial septal defect, high ventricular septal defect, common A-V valve, or clefts in the leaflets of the mitral and tricuspid valves.

Presentation

1. Tachypnea and pallor as a neonate.
2. Common defect in Down's syndrome; examine for other evidence of this condition.
3. Harsh systolic murmur present.
4. Superior electrical axis on ECG.

Treatment. Palliative surgery (pulmonary artery banding) or definitive surgery.

Periductal coarctation syndrome is a form of complex heart disease with no or variable cyanosis in neonates. It is often associated with intracardiac anomalies—VSD, transposition of the great vessels, and aortic valve stenosis. In some forms, the right ventricle may act as the systemic ventricle via a right-to-left shunt at the ductus arteriosus. Treatment is individualized and based on particular hemodynamics.

Massive cardiomegaly in the neonate, with signs of failure and soft or no murmur, may be due to an aberrant left coronary originating from the pulmonary artery; a storage disease such as glucose-6-phosphatase deficiency with massive glycogen deposition in the heart; distal AV fistulae (brain, lungs, liver); endocardial fibroelastosis; or viral myocarditis.

Secundum type atrial septal defect and postductal coarctations of the aorta will only very rarely produce symptoms in infancy.

REFERENCES

See the general list of references following the first section of this chapter.

PATENT DUCTUS ARTERIOSUS

GENERAL CONSIDERATIONS

The ductus arteriosus normally closes within 24 to 48 hrs after birth in the full term infant, but the incidence of PDA increases in inverse proportion to gestational age. The problem is accentuated by modern intensive care through the salvage of very LBW infants, particularly those with respiratory distress. The presence of severe and prolonged lung disease alters the hemodynamics of the pulmonary circulation and tissue oxygenation, both of which adversely affect spontaneous closure of the ductus.

The incidence of a PDA is estimated to be about 35% of all infants weighing less than 1500 g at birth and more than 50% of infants weighing less than 1000 g. A low PaO_2 and prostaglandins of the E type influence patency in utero, and change in the metabolism of prostaglandins after birth and an increase in PaO_2 appear to be important factors in closure. Structural changes occur with maturation so that the more muscular ductus in the term infant has greater potential for closure.

The definition of pathologic patency in the premature is unclear, and considerable controversy has therefore arisen over preventive and ameliorative measures, particularly daily fluid intake.

HEMODYNAMICS

1. In the fetus and at birth, pulmonary artery pressure and pulmonary vascular resistance are high, with a resultant R→L shunt.
2. After birth, as PaO_2 increases and pulmonary artery pressure drops, the R→L shunt decreases.
3. If the ductus remains patent over several days, aortic pressure exceeds pulmonary artery pressure and the shunt becomes L→R.
4. If pulmonary artery pressure remains elevated and the ductus remains large, there may be a bidirectional shunt.
5. With a L→R shunt the left ventricular output increases with a large pulse pressure and resulting decreased or reversed aortic flow during diastole ("aortic steal").

PRESENTATION

Most infants presenting with a PDA in the first weeks of life will be premature, the more immature infants having concomitant HMD. The murmur may be heard intermittently over the first 3–4 days after birth and usually does not become significant until the second week of life, although a patent ductus may not become hemodynamically significant until several weeks of age in a convalescing infant. Most often infants will have a protracted course of respiratory distress requiring mechanical ventilation beyond the first week of life, as well as early signs of bronchopulmonary dysplasia (BPD).

DIAGNOSIS

1. History of concurrent or past HMD or BPD.
2. Murmur:
   a. May vary with the degree and direction of flow.
   b. Best heard over left upper sternal border down LSB.
   c. Continuous murmur not common in premature infants.
   d. Murmur usually pansystolic and harsh, but in prematures it may only be midsystolic.
   e. Heard over back and axilla.
3. Hyperactive precordium.
4. Pulse bounding or accentuated, with easily palpable dorsalis pedis pulse.
5. Heart failure—tachycardia, tachypnea, gallop rhythm. High output failure occurs late with left ventricular overload, hepatomegaly, and pulmonary congestion.
6. Worsening or unresolving pulmonary disease without overt signs of failure.
7. Chest radiograph—cardiomegaly and increased pulmonary vascular markings.
8. Electrocardiogram—no change early, may develop RVH or combined ventricular hypertrophy after several weeks.
9. Echocardiogram—large left atrium and left ventricle. Increased left atrial to aortic dimension ratio (LA/Ao:1.0). Decreased left ventricle pre-ejection to left ventricle ejection time ratio.
10. Heart catheterization seldom necessary or indicated.

THERAPY

1. Restrict fluid intake to <150 mL/kg/day.
2. Diuretics and digoxin may be used if signs of failure (including pulmonary congestion and gallop rhythm) develop. The effi-

cacy of digoxin has not been proved or well tested in prematures with PDA.

3. Maintain hematocrit level above 30%.
4. Indomethacin:
   a. Appears to be more effective during the first 10 days of life.
   b. Dose varies. Twenty-fold variation in plasma indomethacin levels 24 hr after a single dose.
      i. Dosage is 0.2 mg/kg orally, repeat ×3 in 24 hr. IV indomethacin may be more effective, but it is unavailable at present.
      ii. May need more than 1 trial.
      iii. Measure platelet count.
      iv. Determine serum creatinine before, during, and after indomethacin treatment.
      v. Measure plasma indomethacin levels if possible.
5. Surgical ligation is indicated if medical treatment fails or indomethacin is contraindicated. A worsening clinical condition, including increased oxygen needs or increased mechanical ventilation, also requires surgical intervention.

ADDITIONAL COMMENTS

The efficacy of diuretics and the timing and dosages of indomethacin therapy are matters of some controversy. There is also much debate over the role of early closure of a PDA in preventing BPD.

REFERENCES

1. Brash AR, Hickey DE, Graham TP, Stahlman MT, Oates JA, Cotton RB: Pharmacokinetics of indomethacin in the neonate—relation of plasma indomethacin levels to response of the ductus arteriosus. N Eng J Med 305:67, 1981.
2. Gentile R, Stevenson JG, Dooley T, et al: Pulsed Doppler echocardiographic determination of time of ductal closure in normal newborn infants. J Pediatr 98:443, 1981.
3. Siassi B, Blanco C, Cabal LA, Goran AG: Incidence and clinical features of patent ductus arteriosus in low birth weight infants: A prospective analysis of 150 consecutively born infants. Pediatrics 57:347, 1976.
4. Stevenson JG: Fluid administration in the association of patent ductus arteriosus complicating respiratory distress syndrome. J Pediatr 90:257, 1977.
5. White RD, Lietman PS: Commentary: A reappraisal of digitalis for infants with left-to-right shunts and "heart failure." J Pediatr 92:867, 1978.

PERSISTENT FETAL CIRCULATION

GENERAL CONSIDERATIONS

Definition

Persistent fetal circulation (PFC) produces severe hypoxemia in the newborn because there is persistence of right-to-left shunting through fetal channels secondary to elevated pulmonary vascular resistance, sometimes mimicking structural heart disease, sometimes associated with meconium aspiration, and almost always following a prenatal or intrapartum asphyxial event.

Pathogenesis

Vasoconstriction of muscular pulmonary arteries occurs in the fetus. Fetal hypoxia may result in muscular hyperplasia of the pulmonary arterioles. At birth, these vessels may be unusually sensitive to hypoxic or other stimuli and may remain constricted. PFC has also been described following exposure of the fetus to indomethacin (closure of the ductus in utero).

More acute hypoxic distress as might occur with hyaline membrane disease may also result in persistence of fetal shunts.

Pathophysiology

1. Failure of the normal dilatation of the pulmonary vasculature after birth.
2. Persistence of high pulmonary artery pressure and R→L shunting of blood through a PDA.
3. Consequent elevation of right ventricular and right atrial pressures and decreased pulmonary venous return resulting in R→L shunting across the foramen ovale.
4. "Myocardial dysfunction" may accompany PFC owing to increased workload on the right ventricle, tricuspid insufficiency, reduced right coronary artery blood flow, or myocardial ischemia and hypoxia.
5. Persistent hypoxia potentiates the patency of the ductus arteriosus.

PRESENTATION

PFC usually occurs in full term infants who appear profoundly ill following a complicated pregnancy, labor, or delivery. Often there will be evidence of fetal distress; such evidence includes fetal heart rate abnormalities, meconium staining of amniotic fluid, decreased fetal movement, and low 1 and 5 min Apgar scores.

Mildly premature infants (34–38 weeks) with severe hypoxia or HMD probably have some degree of pulmonary hypertension, occasionally severe enough to produce PFC.

The infant usually has respiratory distress characterized by tachypnea with minimal retractions and marked cyanosis, and is often "depressed" or demonstrating signs of previous asphyxia. Heart sounds may be faint. A systolic heart murmur due to tricuspid insufficiency is often heard at lower LSB; a gallop rhythm and narrow splitting of P_2 may also be heard. Systemic arterial pressure may be reduced if myocardial dysfunction is present. Hypovolemia, hypotension, oliguria, and congenital heart failure can occur.

DIAGNOSIS

History. High-risk pregnancy, fetal distress, low Apgar score, and meconium staining with or without aspiration.

Clinical. As above.

Laboratory Assessment

1. Chest radiographs may show clear lung fields with decreased pulmonary vascular markings. Depending on myocardial function, pulmonary venous congestion may develop. There can also be varying degrees of parenchymal changes (HMD, meconium aspiration).
2. PaO_2 less than 60 mm Hg while breathing 100% O_2.
3. Right radial artery to aortic (umbilical artery) differential of PaO_2.
4. Differential of $P_{tc}O_2$ above and below distribution of preductal arterial supply.
5. Electrocardiogram is usually normal, occasionally showing RVH or RVH and LVH. But a hypoxic myocardium may induce development of ST and T wave changes.
6. Doppler echocardiogram confirms R→L shunting through ductus arteriosus and foramen ovale and rules out other structural heart disease. Systolic time intervals assist in evaluating myocardial function.
7. Heart catheterization is indicated if structural heart disease cannot be ruled out by echocardiography.

THERAPY

1. Improve oxygenation:
   a. Increase fractional inspired oxygen concentration (FIO_2) to 100% to maintain $PaO_2 > 50$ mm Hg.

b. Mechanical ventilation:
   i. Hyperventilation ($PaCO_2$ 28–32 mm Hg) to enhance pulmonary vasodilation (not of proven benefit).
   ii. Do not use PEEP levels above 3–4 cm H_2O in absence of parenchymal lung disease.
   iii. Muscle relaxation with pancuronium may be necessary in larger infants. We administer morphine when an infant is paralyzed.

2. Pulmonary vasodilation:
   a. Hyperventilation.
   b. Tolazoline (α-sympathetic blocker) can be used if $PaO_2 < 50$ mm Hg with FIO_2 of 1.0. An IV dose of 1–2 mg/kg is administered into the superior vena caval system over 5–10 min. It may be repeated at 2 mg/kg if there is no response; then administer a continuous infusion of 1–3 mg/kg/hr if no adverse response occurs. Since tolazoline causes general vasodilatation, a fall in systemic arterial pressure often occurs. Therefore, administration of a cardiotonic drug (dopamine) is usually required shortly after tolazoline infusion. There is often an erratic and unpredictable response to this agent.
   c. Other potential vasodilators such as prostaglandin I_2 (prostacyclin) and nifedipine, a calcium channel blocker, may be useful therapeutically but require further testing prior to clinical use. At present, they cannot be recommended.
3. Dopamine—as above. It should be prepared for IV infusion prior to administration of tolazoline. Begin with 2–5 mcg/kg/min and titrate with blood pressure to a maximum dose of 15–20 mcg/kg/min.
4. Alkalosis induced by hyperventilation or infusion of $NaHCO_3$ to reduce pulmonary vasoconstriction is sometimes useful but requires further investigation.
5. Metabolic homeostasis—maintain hematocrit level above 30%, prevent hypoglycemia and hypocalcemia, and minimize oxygen needs.
6. Treat any underlying disease.

ADDITIONAL COMMENTS

1. PFC has a greater than 50% mortality rate.
2. Resolution may occur 36 hr to several weeks after birth, suggesting that supportive care should not be withdrawn if oxygenation is acceptable albeit marginal.
3. Long term follow-up awaits further information:
   a. No cardiopulmonary abnormalities are apparent in the first year of life.
   b. The long term neuro-intellectual outcome is not known, since PFC is a recently recognized syndrome.

REFERENCES

1. Levin DL: Primary pulmonary hypoplasia. J Pediatr 95:550, 1979.
2. Levin DL, Heymann MA, Kitterman JA: Persistent pulmonary hypertension of the newborn infant. J Pediatr 89:626, 1976.
3. Peckham GJ, Fox WW: Physiologic factors affecting pulmonary artery pressure in infants with persistent pulmonary hypertension. J Pediatr 93:1005, 1978.
4. Riemenschneider TA, Nielsen HC, Ruttenberg HD: Disturbances of transitional circulation: spectrum of pulmonary hypertension and myocardial dysfunction. J Pediatr 89:622, 1976.

12

GASTROINTESTINAL DISORDERS

INTESTINAL OBSTRUCTIONS AND BLEEDING

GENERAL CONSIDERATIONS

1. Recognition of the possibility of obstruction and/or perforation at some point along the intestinal tract and institution of appropriate supportive care are more critical than attempting to make a specific anatomic diagnosis of the exact location of the problem.
2. The cardinal signs of gastrointestinal tract obstruction are regurgitation or vomiting of bilious material and abdominal distention. The passage of abnormal-appearing stools, or their absence, is less helpful in arriving at the correct diagnosis.
3. Both the time of onset of symptoms after birth and the degree of abdominal distention will be determined by the level of obstruction.
4. Some obstructions are partial, and symptoms may be intermittent, making it difficult to distinguish a mechanical problem from other causes of feeding difficulty.
5. An intestinal tract obstructed by twisting upon itself (volvulus) can become thickly edematous. Further, any ruptured viscus will be associated with substantial free fluid as well as free air in the peritoneal space. Therefore, the infant suspected of an obstruction or perforation needs extremely close monitoring of blood pressure, pulse rate, and peripheral perfusion to detect early signs of hypovolemic shock. Generous fluid replacement is indicated when intraperitoneal fluid losses are suspected. Some infants, already critically ill on presentation, may benefit from a catheter placed via the saphenous or jugular vein into the right atrium for measuring central venous pressure. Surgery without prior fluid restoration may increase the chances of anesthetic complications.
6. Most conditions—except for volvulus with bowel strangulation—are not emergent. With institution of decompression of the intestinal tract, diagnosis and transfer can proceed in an orderly way.

PRESENTATION AND DIAGNOSIS OF OBSTRUCTIVE LESIONS

1. Bilious vomiting is frequently the first clinical sign of obstruction.
2. Abdominal distention occurs if distal intestine (ileum or colon) is involved. Infants with proximal obstruction (duodenum) are unlikely to have distention, at least early in the course. Duodenal obstruction is likely to be associated with other anomalies, especially Down's syndrome, and may coexist with other intestinal tract abnormalities.
3. Infants may demonstrate signs of discomfort with irritability, crying, and drawing up the legs when the abdomen is palpated.
4. Polyhydramnios, or a history of excessive quantities of fluid (more than 30 mL) retained in the stomach at birth, is strongly suggestive of high intestinal obstruction.
5. Perforation and peritonitis will cause generalized tenderness and blue or purple discoloration of the abdominal wall. The latter sign may be difficult to differentiate from local hemorrhage into the tissues of the abdominal wall. Such a hemorrhage may occur with any bleeding disorder, including disseminated intravascular coagulation (DIC). However, intestinal ischemic lesions themselves may produce DIC and generalized bleeding.
6. Changes in abdominal sounds are less reliable in the newborn. Bowel sounds may be present no matter what type of lesion has occurred, although persistent peritonitis will usually produce ileus and a "silent" abdomen.
7. Passage of meconium stools does not eliminate the diagnostic possibility of an obstruction. Failure to pass any meconium may suggest the presence of Hirschsprung's disease.
8. The initial diagnostic study should be to obtain abdominal radiographs, including both supine and upright or lateral views. Radiographic signs of obstruction include a thickened bowel wall, distended loops with multiple air-fluid levels, absence of air in the rectum, and "double bubble." Free peritoneal air is found when a perforation has occurred.
9. Rectal examination with the finger may be of use in the diagnostic evaluation, if a mass is felt. This may indicate the presence of an abscess secondary to an appendiceal perforation.

TYPES OF OBSTRUCTION

1. *Malrotation* (technically nonrotation) occurs because of inadequate fixation of the intestinal mesentery as the intestine returns to the abdominal cavity during fetal development. This results in inappropriate location of the midgut, especially the

cecum. Bands form between the ectopically-located cecum and the abdominal wall. These bands may partially compress the duodenum, producing a high and sometimes intermittent obstruction.

2. *Volvulus* occurs with malrotation when the intestine twists on the axis of the superior mesenteric artery, producing obstruction and ischemia.
3. *Duodenal obstruction* may occur because of an intrinsic defect (stenosis or atresia) or because the hollow tube is compressed by an annular pancreas. Abdominal radiographs will show the double bubble sign—air in the stomach and proximal duodenum, with no distal bowel gas.
4. *Jejunal atresia* manifests itself later after birth than duodenal atresia. The abdominal radiograph will show multiple air-fluid levels, as opposed to the typical two air bubbles of distal duodenal atresia.
5. Rare causes of intestinal obstruction include *duplications* or *cysts* that may form anywhere along the gastrointestinal tract and, when distended, block the normal peristaltic advancement of intraluminal fluids.
6. *Meconium ileus* occurs in infants genetically predisposed to develop cystic fibrosis. The ileus occurs when thick viscous meconium obstructs the distal small intestine and the cecum. Abdominal radiographic examination of the right lower quadrant demonstrates a nondescript mass, sometimes with calcifications, and a paucity of air-fluid levels on the upright view because of the viscous intrabdominal contents. Barium studies will show a diffusely small colon. Prenatal perforation may have occurred and will be detectable by the presence of calcifications in the peritoneal space. Such calcifications can be seen radiographically. Relief of obstruction may be obtained by rectal instillation of saline or hyperosmolar agents, *but* there is a risk of intravascular fluid depletion and shock with this therapy. Infants with meconium ileus should be assumed to have cystic fibrosis. The diagnosis can be confirmed as early as several weeks of age by sweat chloride analysis; analyses of stool enzymes and serum immunoreactive enzymes have a high incidence of false negative results in infants with meconium ileus.
7. *Hirschsprung's disease* is manifested by failure of intrinsic peristalsis in the colon because of a lack of neuroganglion tissue in bowel wall segments, producing complete or, more commonly, intermittent obstruction. Rarely, this condition produces life-threatening complications (toxic megacolon and enterocolitis) in the first days of life. Emergency treatment consists of intravascular fluid replacement, antibiotics, abdominal decompression, and colostomy in a segment of ganglionic bowel proximal to the aganglionic segment.

8. *Imperforate anus* is a rare cause of obstruction. It is usually associated with other, more obvious congenital anomalies of the cardiac, gastrointestinal, and especially genitourinary systems. A fistula between the distal intestinal tract and the genitourinary tract is present in both sexes. The life-threatening aspect of this anomaly usually arises from the associated malformations.

GASTROINTESTINAL BLEEDING

Gastrointestinal bleeding in newborns—unlike bleeding in adults—is rarely an emergency when the bleeding occurs in what appears to be an otherwise healthy patient. The physician's first task is to consider and rule out both a generalized bleeding disorder (see Chapter 16) and a generalized disorder of the intestinal tract, especially necrotizing enterocolitis (see section on Necrotizing Enterocolitis, this chapter). Frequently, the blood that is found is maternal blood swallowed by the newborn and therefore of no concern. At least half of the remaining cases are idiopathic and remain undiagnosed. Intermittent vascular compromise to the gut from the volvulus or malrotation with secondary bleeding from ischemic sites is the most feared cause of blood in the stools of newborns and is likely to present with grossly obvious blood in the stool and not simply guaiac-positive stools. Other symptoms—distention, vomiting, or irritability—should be sought and appropriate diagnostic studies undertaken if any question remains about the possibility of this diagnosis. Intussusception is a rare cause of neonatal intestinal bleeding. Meckel's diverticulum, an intestinal malformation containing aberrant gastric tissue, may also occasionally bleed in the newborn period and can be diagnosed by radionuclide scanning techniques.

ADDITIONAL COMMENTS

1. Tracheoesophageal fistulae are discussed in Chapter 9 because of their presentation with respiratory distress.
2. Neonatal appendicitis may not present with clinical findings until rupture and generalized peritonitis have occurred. Because of the absence of the early localizing findings, appendicitis involves a high mortality when it occurs in young infants.
3. Abdominal tumors present in newborns as firm masses, diagnosed only on physical examination. They most commonly produce their effects on the genitourinary (not the gastrointestinal) system by either extrinsic compression (neuroblastoma) or intrinsic interference (Wilms' tumor) with the kidney and ureters. A rapid, orderly diagnostic evaluation precedes sur-

gery. Abdominal ultrasonography can help differentiate the rare nonoperable lesion (adrenal hemorrhage, certain cysts) from the many lesions that will require surgery.

REFERENCES

1. Hendren WH: Pediatric surgery (part II). N Engl J Med 289:507, 1973.
2. Johnson DG: Emergency surgical management of life threatening anomalies in neonates. Hosp Pract, February 1975, p. 69.
3. Koop CE: Abdominal masses in the newborn infant. N Engl J Med 289:569, 1973.

ABDOMINAL WALL ANOMALIES REQUIRING EMERGENCY TREATMENT

GENERAL CONSIDERATIONS

Two major defects are recognized: omphalocele and gastroschisis. Omphalocele results from a first trimester arrest in the closure of the abdominal wall whereby a herniated sac of abdominal contents remains extruded through a defect in the umbilical ring. This extrusion is intimately related to a malplaced umbilicus. Gastroschisis (literally meaning "belly cleft") occurs because of an abdominal wall defect at the base of the normally positioned umbilical stalk, which also results in exterioration of bowel loops. Differentiation of the two lesions can be made if a covering sac is present or if the umbilicus is abnormally positioned. Either indicates that the lesion is an omphalocele. Surgical treatment is mandatory in both cases.

Presentation is at birth or earlier if fetal ultrasound examination is made.

Diagnosis is by inspection. The bowel loops will appear swollen, discolored, and matted with gastroschisis or a long-ruptured omphalocele because of contact with the acidic amniotic fluid.

MANAGEMENT

The physician has several tasks to be performed immediately:

1. Resuscitate the infant if necessary, and dry him.
2. Cover the exposed abdominal contents quickly with *warm sterile* gauze pads soaked in sterile saline. Pads must be *kept* warm and wet. It is preferable also to cover the defect with occlusive plastic to minimize water and heat loss, which can be extensive.
3. Use a large-bore nasogastric tube for continuous suction. Remember to add the extra fluid loss to initial intravenous therapy fluid calculations.

4. Begin intravenous fluid infusion at a generous rate (120–150 mL/kg/24 hr) and follow vital signs and serum electrolytes closely (q 8–12 hr) with the expectation that excessive water and electrolyte loss and eventually intravascular depletion will occur.
5. Turn the baby on his side so the weight of the dressing and abdominal contents will not compromise respiratory efforts.
6. Examine the infant for other signs of congenital anomalies. Infants with omphalocele may have as much as a 50% chance of having associated anomalies. The most likely associated defects usually involve renal or cardiovascular systems. Omphalocele also occurs in trisomy 13 and 18 and in the macrosomia syndrome described by Beckwith. Gastroschisis has a much lower risk of associated anomalies. Detailed knowledge of the presence and extent of such anomalies obviously alters subsequent management.
7. Begin antibiotic therapy for the presumed contamination of bowel and subsequent peritonitis. Suggested treatment is ampicillin and gentamicin to provide broad-spectrum coverage for the wide assortment of potentially contaminating organisms.
8. Arrange surgical consultation, and, if necessary, transport. The risk of infection increases when the bowel contents remain exposed for long periods.

ADDITIONAL COMMENTS

1. The availability of long term, relatively safe parenteral nutrition has allowed many infants with these conditions to survive and live normally.
2. Considerable surgical judgment is required to determine whether primary closure or staged closure of the defect is safer. Prolonged ileus is more likely with gastroschisis. Oral feedings should be withheld following primary closure for a number of days and then started very slowly.

REFERENCES

See the references listed after the section on Gastrointestinal Emergencies.

NECROTIZING ENTEROCOLITIS

GENERAL CONSIDERATIONS

Definition

Necrotizing enterocolitis (NEC) is manifested by necrotic, inflammatory, and hemorrhagic lesions of the mucosa of the small and large bowel; bowel wall perforations; spillage of intestinal contents; and peritonitis.

Mucosal lesions may be scattered throughout the entire length of the intestinal tract, but they most commonly occur in the ileum, with normal intestine interspersed (so-called skip lesions). The disease may produce intramural gas bubbles that are visible radiographically. Incidence of the disease is 4–5% of newborn intensive care unit admissions. Some centers report that 25% of infants of less than 1200 g birth weight are affected by the disease.

Etiology

The disease is probably of multifactorial etiology, with antecedent hypoxic-ischemic injury of the intestinal tract a major component. Normally nonpathogenic bacteria of the intestinal tract may infect the mucosa. These bacteria cause hydrogen gas formation within the bowel wall. Disease onset usually follows milk feedings, which may increase metabolic demands on the already compromised intestinal mucosa.

PRESENTATION

This illness usually affects premature infants less than 3 weeks of age and less than 1500 g birth weight. Usually NEC occurs during the first week of life, but it may occur in very LBW infants up to 2 months of age if they have been severely ill.

The disease is rare in infants fed only fresh breast milk and in infants who have not yet been fed.

The infant usually has had other illnesses—birth asphyxia, hyaline membrane disease, apnea, or jaundice requiring exchange transfusion. There is frequently a history of umbilical artery catheterization.

Signs and Symptoms

Generalized signs include temperature instability, lethargy, and increased apnea.

Signs specific to the intestinal tract include abdominal distention, poor feeding tolerance with regurgitation or residuals of gastric feedings, decreased stools, bloody stools, abdominal tenderness, and lower quadrant mass.

There may be no signs or symptoms referable to the intestinal tract in very LBW infants who have developed the disease.

DIAGNOSIS

Radiographic

The diagnosis is confirmed by abdominal radiographs taken in the upright and supine positions. These may demonstrate free intraperitoneal air if perforation has occurred. They should demonstrate the pattern of pneumatosis intestinalis, most commonly found in the right lower quadrant (distal ileum). Other findings may include free abdominal fluid or a pattern of hepatic portal venous gas.

Other Laboratory Findings

1. Metabolic acidosis is often present.
2. Total leukocyte count and neutrophil count are abnormal. Profound neutropenia or an elevated band count may occur in infants who have acquired a generalized infection with the disease.
3. Absolute thrombocytopenia or a falling platelet count often occurs.
4. Blood and spinal fluid cultures often are positive in NEC.

THERAPY

General

Treat shock, if present, with increased fluids. Carefully monitor blood pressure and urine output.

Treat the infection with broad-spectrum, systemically administered antibiotics, including ampicillin (50 mg/kg q 12 hr for the first week of life, then 50/mg q 8 hr) and gentamicin (2.5 mg/kg q 12 hr for the first week of life, then 2.5 mg/kg q 8 hr). The antibiotic or the dosage may need to be changed according to culture results.

Correct acidosis with an infusion of bicarbonate.

Correct abnormal coagulation status with an infusion of platelet-rich plasma or fresh frozen plasma when coagulation studies so indicate.

Gastrointestinal

The infant should have no oral intake. Decompression of the abdomen is accomplished by placement of a nasogastric tube, and often a gastrostomy tube is placed at surgery.

Indications for surgery, with resection of the involved bowel, are the presence of free air on abdominal radiographs and signs of peritonitis, intestinal obstruction, or deteriorating clinical condition as indicated by increasingly severe metabolic acidosis or progressive thrombocytopenia. Pneumatosis intestinalis alone is not an indication for surgical intervention.

Parenteral alimentation should be instituted if (1) surgery with resection of the small bowel and a colostomy or ileostomy is performed, (2) peritonitis is present, or (3) the infant cannot be fed for several days. This alimentation can be supplied through the peripheral or the central vein.

OUTCOME

1. Immediate survival probability is 67% if surgery is not indicated and 33% if surgery is necessary.
2. Long term problems in survivors may include a small risk of developing strictures at the point of disease or developing adhesions if peritonitis has occurred. In addition, there is a risk of developing malabsorption syndrome if extensive surgical resection of the intestine has been necessary.
3. Surgical reanastomosis of the colostomy or ileostomy is usually performed at 4 to 6 months of age or at a minimum weight of 2500 g.

ADDITIONAL COMMENTS

1. Premature infants frequently have episodes of abdominal distention and feeding intolerance during the first weeks of life. Such infants need to be closely followed to determine if these signs will progress until all the findings of NEC appear. At the least, feedings should be withheld until the distention is resolved.
2. Prophylactic or therapeutic use of enteric antibiotics is of uncertain benefit in NEC.

REFERENCES

1. Hutter JJ, Hathaway WE, Wayne ER: Hematologic abnormalities in severe neonatal necrotizing enterocolitis. J Pediatr 88:1026, 1976.
2. Ross Conference on Pediatric Research, 68: Necrotizing enterocolitis in the newborn infant. 1975.
3. Santulli EV, Schullinger JN, Heird WC, et al: Acute necrotizing enterocolitis in infancy: a review of 64 cases. Pediatrics 55:376, 1975.
4. Stevenson DK, Graham CB, Stevenson JK: Neonatal necrotizing enterocolitis: one hundred new cases. Adv Pediatr 27:319, 1980.

13

METABOLIC AND ENDOCRINE EMERGENCIES

HYPOGLYCEMIA

GENERAL CONSIDERATIONS

Hypoglycemia is defined as a blood glucose level of less than 30 mg/dL. A level of less than 20 mg/dL has been used as a strict definition of hypoglycemia; however, all infants in our Neonatal Intensive Care Unit (NICU) are treated for hypoglycemia if the blood glucose level is less than 30 mg/dL. The overall incidence of hypoglycemia is about 2–3/1000 live births. It occurs more commonly in SGA infants, twins, infants of diabetic mothers (IDM), infants of toxemic mothers, and critically ill infants. Transient hypoglycemia during the first 12 hr of life occurs in approximately 20% of premature infants.

Several categories of hypoglycemia have been described, but the vast majority of cases are transient.

1. *Transient early hypoglycemia* is probably an adaptive phenomenon related to hypothermic stress or an adrenergic influence that could increase glucose utilization. The fetal blood glucose level will reflect the maternal serum glucose concentration, with reactive hypoglycemia occurring in the first 4 hr of life.
2. *Secondary hypoglycemia* is associated with other abnormal conditions such as shock, sepsis, SGA, maternal drugs, maternal diabetes, congenital heart disease, and erythroblastosis.
3. *Persistent severe hypoglycemia* is rare and requires a more extensive evaluation and treatment. Included in this category are Beckwith-Weidemann syndrome, leucine sensitivity, islet cell adenoma, nesidioblastosis, adrenal insufficiency, pituitary-hypothalamic disorders, and enzymatic defects in carbohydrate metabolism.

PRESENTATION

Many infants remain asymptomatic with hypoglycemia, whereas others present with jitteriness, tremors, seizures, apnea, irritability, exaggerated Moro's reflex, hypotonia, limpness, apathy, cyanosis, or tachypnea, usually in the first 48 hr of life. IDM are often asymptomatic in the presence of a low blood glucose level during the first 4–6 hr of life.

Other associated abnormalities may be present, including cardiac enlargement, central nervous system abnormalities, erythroblastosis, cold injury, adrenal hemorrhage, and exchange transfusion.

DIAGNOSIS

History

Check the history of maternal drugs (chlorpropamide, benzothiazide derivatives, salicylates), maternal diabetes, Rh incompatibility, intrauterine growth retardation, fetal asphyxia, and siblings with galactosemia.

Clinical

A physical examination will determine if the infant is SGA, LGA, or postmature or has features of an IDM (see Chapter 19). Macrosomia and protruding tongue are consistent with Beckwith's syndrome. Look for hepatomegaly, genital abnormalities, and other CNS congenital defects.

All premature and critically ill infants are suspect. Color indicators (e.g., Chemstrips) should be used to determine blood glucose levels in all infants with overt signs (e.g., seizures and sudden onset of apnea). Serum calcium levels should also be determined. A prompt response to intravenous 10–15% glucose helps to confirm the diagnosis. Cerebrospinal glucose levels will be low.

Additional studies are indicated to detect underlying disorders in infants with persistent or recurrent hypoglycemia. Determine plasma insulin, free thyroxine (T_4), ketones, pH, lactate, and pyruvate levels, as well as levels of urine amino acids, organic acids, and reducing substances. Pending these results and other physical findings, more definitive tests for glucagon tolerance, cortisol levels, human growth hormone (HGH), and alanine response may be indicated.

TREATMENT

1. Early glucose feeding with milk or D10W for infants at risk.
2. IV D10W for asphyxiated, extremely LBW, or at-risk infants.
3. Symptomatic hypoglycemia: IV D10W, IVDION, giving at least 5–7 mg/kg body weight by infusing of 1–2 mL/min, followed by a slow infusion of D10W at 4–8 mg/kg/min.
4. Some infants may require D15W or even higher concentrations, depending on the cause of hypoglycemia.

5. Because the underlying metabolic rate and the remaining stores of glucose are unknown, it is difficult to arrive at a single dose of glucose adequate for all situations, yet not producing sudden hyperglycemia and osmolality changes.
6. Glucagon should only be administered just prior to neonatal transport or if IV glucose cannot be administered.
7. If intractable (i.e., after 72 hours), add glucocorticoid:

Hydrocortisone or	5 mg/kg/day intramuscularly q 12 hr
Solu-Cortef or	5 mg/kg/day intravenously q 6 hr
Prednisone	2 mg/kg/day orally

   Surgery with removal of 80–90% of pancreas may be necessary for hyperinsulinemic conditions. Diazoxide is not recommended for control of hypoglycemia.
8. Wean by reducing IV dose slowly (e.g., from 8–10 mg/kg/min to 4 mg/kg/min) while increasing oral feedings.
9. Avoid peripheral vein utilization when concentrations ⩾D15W are needed.

ADDITIONAL COMMENTS

1. The long term consequences of transient hypoglycemia appear to be minimal. Neurologic sequelae may be related to an association between CNS dysfunction at birth and resultant hypoglycemia.
2. Some controversy exists over the necessity of treating asymptomatic hypoglycemia, particularly in IDM. We favor glucose therapy for all infants with documented hypoglycemia.

REFERENCES

1. Cornblath M, Schwartz R (eds): Hypoglycemia in the Neonate. *In* Disorders of Carbohydrate Metabolism in Infancy, 2nd ed. Philadelphia, Saunders, 1976, p. 155.
2. deLeeuw R, deVries IJ: Hypoglycemia in small for dates newborn infants. Pediatrics 58:18, 1976.
3. Gatbeittet RL, Cornblath M: Neonatal hypoglycemia revisited, 1975. Pediatrics 58:1, 1976.
4. Senior B: Current concepts. Neonatal hypoglycemia. N Engl J Med 289:790, 1973.
5. Shelley HJ, Bassett JM: Control of carbohydrate metabolism in the fetus and newborn. Br Med Bull 31:37, 1975.
6. Søvik O, Vidnes J, Walkner S: Persistent neonatal hypoglycemia. Acta Pathol Microbiol Scand 83(Section A):155, 1975.

HYPOCALCEMIA

GENERAL CONSIDERATIONS

Hypocalcemia is defined as a serum calcium level of less than 7.0 mg/dL or an ionized calcium level of less than 3.5 mg/dL. The incidence is approximately one third of all premature infants, one third of asphyxiated infants, and approximately one half of infants of insulin-dependent diabetic mothers.

PATHOPHYSIOLOGY

Fetal parathyroid function begins in the second trimester, but its functions are influenced by the transplacental movement of maternal calcium ions. Maternal parathyroid activity is normally high at birth and produces a high fetal serum calcium level. After birth, there is an abrupt decrease in calcium intake, particularly in the sick infant. A state of functional hypoparathyroidism exists. The premature infant has a greater degree of functional hypoparathyroidism, characterized by increased endogenous phosphorus production (due to increased glycogen breakdown and decreased renal excretion of phosphorus), decreased calcium intake, and decreased circulating vitamin D metabolites. Calcitonin, produced in the thyroid gland, inhibits bone resorption and has a calciuric effect. Following birth, there is a physiologic increase in calcitonin, further increased by hypoxia, and this may contribute to the common occurrence of hypocalcemia; however, this would not explain the phosphatemia associated with hypocalcemia. Etiologic factors include prematurity, birth asphyxia, intrauterine growth retardation, diabetic mothers, exchange transfusion, treatment of metabolic acidosis with sodium bicarbonate, and free fatty acid infusion during total parenteral nutrition.

PRESENTATION

Hypocalcemia usually occurs during the first 72 hr of life and most infants are asymptomatic. However, infants may demonstrate evidence of hyperactivity, irritability, jitteriness, and seizures that may be associated with cyanosis. Relief of signs will occur on injection of calcium gluconate intravenously.

Late hypocalcemia, or classic neonatal tetany, occurs about 6 or 7 days after birth and is associated with a high phosphorus intake and hyperphosphatemia. This form of hypocalcemia is extremely rare, since commercial formulas no longer provide an excess of phosphorus and have a calcium-phosphorus ratio closer to that of breast milk.

LABORATORY

1. The total serum (bound) calcium level is less than 7.0 mg/dL.
2. The ionized calcium level is less than 3.5 mg/dL. The blood sample must be obtained anaerobically by venipuncture for ionized calcium determination.
3. The $Q\text{-}_0T_c$ interval (from the beginning of the QRS complex to the origin of the T wave on the ECG, corrected for rate) is unreliable. Although there is some correlation with hypocalcemia, it has not proved to be an accurate diagnostic tool.
4. A serum phosphorus level greater than 8 mg/dL and a serum magnesium level of less than 1.5 mg/dL are abnormal.

THERAPY

Symptomatic Hypocalcemia

Administer 10% calcium gluconate 1–2 mL/kg/10 min while monitoring the electrocardiogram continuously.

Asymptomatic Hypocalcemia

Administer an intravenous infusion of 50 mg elemental calcium/kg/day as calcium gluconate or gluceptate. Controversy exists over the efficacy of continuous versus intermittent calcium infusions.

One mL of 10% calcium gluconate contains 100 mg of calcium gluconate or 9 mg of elemental calcium. One mL of calcium gluceptate contains 18 mg of elemental calcium.

These infusions should not be mixed with sodium bicarbonate. If a continuous infusion of calcium is used, it is important to clear the intravascular catheter thoroughly of infusate before administering bicarbonate.

Note of caution: rapid infusion of calcium can result in a cardiac arrest.

Oral Therapy

Some recommend the enteric administration of calcium salts in the form of 75 mg/kg/day of elemental calcium divided into six doses. There is some controversy over the use of oral calcium owing to a possible increased risk of necrotizing enterocolitis.

ADDITIONAL COMMENTS

1. Magnesium metabolism is closely related to calcium metabolism. Hypomagnesemia may be associated with hypocalcemia

and can influence parathyroid hormone function. Low magnesium levels also need treatment with a dose of 0.1–0.2 mL/kg of 50% magnesium sulfate. It is necessary to monitor serum levels.

2. If persistent hypocalcemia occurs, a more extensive evaluation is indicated to determine if there is an abnormal renal loss of calcium or an altered vitamin D metabolism.
3. Oral dietary supplementation with vitamin D is recommended to prevent rickets, especially in premature infants. See Chapter 8, Neonatal Nutrition, for dosage.

REFERENCES

1. Brown D, Salsbury D: Short term biochemical effects of parenteral calcium treatment of early onset neonatal hypocalcemia. J Pediatr 100:777, 1982.
2. Brown D, Steranka B, Taylor F: Treatment of early onset of neonatal hypocalcemia. Amer J Dis Child 135:24, 1981.
3. Tsang RC, Chen I, Atkinson W, Hayes W, Athenton H, Edwards N: Neonatal hypocalcemia in birth asphyxia. J Pediatr 84:428, 1974.
4. Tsang RC, Chen IN, Thiedman MA, Chen I: Neonatal parathyroid function; role of gestational and postnatal age. J Pediatr 83:728, 1973.

THYROID GLAND DISORDERS

GENERAL CONSIDERATIONS

The thyroid gland begins to function after 12 weeks of fetal life. Thyrotropin (TSH) and thyroxine (T_4) increase after mid-gestation, and the fetus develops a functioning hypothalamic-pituitary-thyroid axis that is independent of the mother's thyroid function. By 26 weeks' gestation, TSH exceeds maternal levels and T_4 synthesis and secretions are TSH-dependent. T_4 does not appear to be essential to fetal growth. The placenta is impermeable to TSH, T_4, and triiodothyroxine (T_3), so maternal serum levels are unrelated to fetal levels. Maternal iodide, propylthiouracil (PTU), and long-acting thyroid stimulator (LATS), however, can cross the placenta and seriously affect fetal thyroid development and function. T_3 levels are lower in the fetus than in the mother, whereas reverse T_3 levels are elevated. Fetal thyroxine-binding globulin (TBG) levels increase during the last half of gestation.

Released T_4 is bound to 3 proteins in the plasma: 75% is bound to TBG, 15% to thyroxine-binding prealbumin (TBPA), and 10% to serum albumin. Free T_4 is the biologically active fraction, subsequent to peripheral deiodination.

There is a surge in TSH and T_4 immediately after birth as a normal part of successful adaptation to extrauterine life. At birth the umbilical cord T_4 level is approximately 12±4 (standard deviation) μg/dL. Within a few minutes of birth there is a marked rise in TSH to a maximum level of about 100 μU/mL, probably related to body temperature changes. The TSH level subsequently decreases over the next 24–72 hr. T_4 levels peak by about 48 hr at 15–20 μg/dL, indicating that a state of physiologic hyperthyroidism normally exists for the first 1–2 days. T_4 levels remain high for about 2 weeks, dropping to 8–10 μg/dL by 4–6 weeks of life.

The premature infant has a lower level of T_4 correlating directly with gestational age. In addition, the presence of intercurrent illness, particularly respiratory distress, can result in depressed T_4 levels. Premature infants also have decreased levels of albumin, TBG, and other serum proteins, which make for low T_4 levels. Protein levels may be further depressed in the presence of critical illness.

CONGENITAL HYPOTHYROIDISM

1. Thyrotropin releasing hormone (TRH) deficiency is associated with a variety of congenital defects.
2. TSH deficiency is sometimes associated with other pituitary gland defects.
3. Etiology of thyroid hormone deficiency:
   a. Athyreosis or dysgenesis.
   b. Inborn errors of synthesis (includes several defects).
   c. Iodine deficiency.
   d. Maternal thyroiditis—antibodies.
   e. Maternal drugs—PTU, iodides, lithium.
4. TSH unresponsiveness.
5. T_4 unresponsiveness.

Presentation

Usually no obvious signs occur until several weeks of life. Early manifestations of hypothyroidism include lethargy, hypotonia, poor feeding, weak sucking, mottling, a hoarse cry, jaundice, decreased core temperature, large anterior and posterior fontanels, and a protruding tongue. Delays in motor development, poor growth, listlessness, and constipation are signs that usually appear later.

Diagnosis

$T_4 < 6 \mu g$/dL at 3 days of age (normal range 8–15). TSH > 20 μU/mL beyond 3 days (normal 5–20).

Note: avoid testing during first 3 days of life owing to surge in TSH and T_4 at birth. Zero radioactive iodine uptake will confirm athyreosis, or uptake by technetium scan will detect the presence of thyroid tissue. (These tests are usually not very reliable.)

Treatment

Synthetic levothyroxine sodium provides both T_4 and T_3 in an oral dose of 25–50 μg/day. The dose should be gradually increased over the first year of life to approximately 100 μg/day.

HYPERTHYROIDISM

The fetal thyroid may be stimulated by transplacental long-acting thyroid stimulator (LATS) in mothers with active or past Graves' disease. This occurrence is rare, however, since thyrotoxic women do not often complete a pregnancy. Serum LATS will gradually decrease after birth with an estimated half-life of 20 days.

Presentation

Neonatal thyrotoxicosis may present within the first 24 hr of life and is characterized by increased activity, tachycardia, sweating, irritability, and hyperthermia. Subsequent signs are increased appetite, poor weight gain, and minimal exophthalmos. The thyroid may be palpable and increase in size after birth. In severe cases arrhythmias and heart failure may ensue. If antithyroid drugs have been given to the mother, there may be no evidence of hyperthyroidism during the first several days of life. However, since the serum LATS persists for a much longer time than antithyroid drugs, the onset of symptoms may be delayed for several days.

Diagnosis

1. Maternal history of Graves' disease.
2. Treatment of mother with antithyroid drugs.
3. Serial palpation of thyroid gland.
4. T_4 and free T_4 on 2 or 3 occasions serially in the first 10 days.
5. Serum level of LATS in mother, umbilical cord blood, and baby.

Therapy

Serial examination of serum LATS will help determine the length of treatment, which should be several weeks. Antithyroid drugs may include PTU, Lugol's iodine, methimazole, and propranolol:

PTU	10 mg/kg/day q 8 hr.
Methimazole	0.5–1.0 mg/kg/day q 8 hr.

Lugol's iodine	1 drop tid, may need to increase dose if there is no response or effects disappear
Propranolol	2 mg/kg/day bid may be indicated to decrease adrenergic effects
Digitalis	Should be administered if there are signs of cardiac failure (see dosage in Table 20–6).

REFERENCES

1. Cuestas RA: Thyroid function in healthy premature infants. J Pediatr 92:963, 1978.
2. Fisher DA, Burrow GN (eds): Perinatal Thyroid Physiology and Disease. New York, Raven Press, 1975.
3. Fisher DA, Klein AH: Thyroid development and disorders of thyroid development and disorders of thyroid function in the newborn. N Engl J Med 304:702, 1981.
4. Hadeed AJ, Asay LD, Klein AH et al: Significance of transient postnatal hypothyroxinemia in premature infants with and without respiratory distress syndrome. Pediatrics 68:464, 1981.
5. Oddie TH, Fisher DA, Bernard B et al: Thyroid function at birth in infants of 30–45 weeks' gestation. J Pediatr 90:803, 1977.
6. Redmond GP: Therapy of congenital hypothyroidism in the era of mass screening. Semin Perinatol 6:181, 1982.

AMBIGUOUS GENITALIA

GENERAL CONSIDERATIONS

Disorders of sexual differentiation producing ambiguous genitalia may result from a variety of causes. Abnormal development can occur at various stages of fetal differentiation and cause various malformations. It is urgent to decide the gender assignment as quickly as possible to ease parental anxiety and plan appropriate treatment. Gender assignment and sex rearing should be determined more by anatomic aspects than by genotype, since gonadal genotype is not critical to psychosexual male or female expression.

It is important to understand the sexual development of common fetal gonads and internal structures. The female phenotype will develop unless opposed by male sex chromosomes. Hormonal secretion by fetal testes inhibits müllerian duct formation, and androgen secretion stimulates mesonephric duct development. Normal differentiation is completed during the first trimester.

Etiology

1. Female pseudohermaphroditism (masculinization):
   a. Adrenogenital syndrome.

   b. Drug-induced.
   c. Androgen-producing tumors in mother.
   d. Idiopathic.
   e. Part of a more complex congenital defect (e.g., CHARGE association: colobomata, heart defect, atresia of the choanae, retardation of growth, genital hypoplasia, and ear anomalies).
2. Male pseudohermaphroditism (incomplete masculinization):
   a. Testicular deficiencies:
      i. Leydig's cell aplasia.
      ii. Abnormal differentiation—gonadal agenesis or dysgenesis.
   b. Testosterone deficiencies:
      i. Synthetic defects (adrenogenital syndrome).
      ii. Conversion defect.
   c. Associated with Wilms' tumor.
3. True hermaphroditism (XX, XY, XX/XY, familial).

PRESENTATION

The external genitalia may vary in appearance from cryptorchidism with a normal phallus to severe hypospadias. The phallus may be of a normal male size, but it often appears as an enlarged clitoris. Gonads may be palpable in the inguinal canal. Scrotal folds may appear as fused labia majora. The urethral opening may be on the dorsal side of the phallus or penoscrotal. Often other congenital malformations are present.

DIAGNOSIS

1. Historical:
   a. Deaths among previously born infants.
   b. History of males with hypospadias or cryptorchidism.
   c. Maternal drug exposure (progestogens, phenytoin).
2. Clinical:
   a. Palpate to determine presence, site, and size of gonads. A palpable inguinal gonad indicates a male genotype. (Very rarely, one inguinal gonad indicates a true hermaphrodite.)
   b. Determine phallus size.
   c. Note site of urethral opening.
   d. Look for other anomalies.

Other Studies

1. Buccal smear.
2. Chromosomal analysis—bone marrow aspiration should provide information in 24–48 hr.

3. Rule out congenital adrenal hyperplasia by serum or urinary 17-alpha-hydroxy-progesterone or by urinary 17-ketosteroid elevation. Salt-losing forms may present by the end of the first week of life, so serial electrolytes, blood pressure, and urine output are important to monitor.
4. Sinograms of the urethral orifice.
5. Ultrasonography for the presence of a uterus and gonads.

MANAGEMENT

1. Do not circumcise.
2. Have a urologic surgeon determine time and need for future reconstructive surgery.
3. Counsel parents (definitive diagnosis usually takes 1 week), and coordinate consultants (urologist, psychologist, geneticist).
4. Repeat buccal smear after the third day because of a 25% incidence of false-negative on the first day.
5. If the adrenogenital syndrome is diagnosed, human leukocyte antigen (HLA) typing of the infant is important because of the linkage between 21-hydroxylase deficiency and HLA type. This may allow for prenatal diagnosis in a later pregnancy.
6. Exploratory laparotomy, if necessary, should be delayed beyond the neonatal period.
7. Likewise delay laparoscopy.

ADDITIONAL COMMENTS

All discussions with the parents should be coordinated through a single responsible physician to minimize parental anxieties and confusion. This should obviate some of the sense of urgency and allow an efficient and complete evaluation to proceed in an orderly fashion.

14

INFECTIOUS DISORDERS

INTRODUCTION

Bacterial sepsis, typically acquired during or shortly after birth, affects 1 in 2000 full term infants, 1 in 200 infants of birth weight less than 2500 g, and 1 in 10 infants of birth weight less than 1000 g. Twenty to 30% develop concomitant meningitis; 20-50% die, depending on coexisting conditions and the etiologic agent. Many of the survivors of combined sepsis and meningitis are cursed with crippling permanent neurologic sequelae. Intensive care units have failed to diminish either the incidence or, surprisingly, the morbidity of these infections. The clustering of many critically ill infants in crowded nurseries may enhance the risk of bacterial infection.

Exhaustive and elaborate attempts have been made to devise accurate and sensitive clinical and laboratory indices to identify infants likely to have sepsis. None of these attempts has been totally successful, and clinical judgment remains paramount in the diagnosis of sepsis.

There are many reasons for the increased susceptibility of the newborn to widespread bacterial infection. These include mechanical factors (such as increased skin fragility and development of pulmonary atelectasis) and immunologic factors (such as depressed function of neutrophils, lack of prior exposure to illness, and dependence of the fetal antibody spectrum upon that received from the mother).

BACTERIAL SEPSIS AND MENINGITIS

MOST COMMON ETIOLOGIC AGENTS

In most nurseries in North America, *Escherichia coli* and Group B Streptococcus together account for about 70% of all infections. The physician must remember that enterovirus and perhaps CMV also can produce a constellation of signs clinically similar to those produced by the organisms listed in Table 14–1.

PREDISPOSING RISK FACTORS

1. Premature delivery.
2. Prolonged rupture of membranes (defined variously as prior to onset of labor or as more than 24 hr prior to delivery). The

Table 14–1. ETIOLOGIC AGENTS OF NEONATAL BACTERIAL SEPSIS

GRAM-POSITIVE ORGANISMS	GRAM-NEGATIVE ORGANISMS
Group B Streptococcus	*Escherichia coli*
Group D Streptococcus (*Streptococcus faecalis*)	Pseudomonas species
Streptococcus pneumoniae	*Proteus mirabilis*
Listeria monocytogenes	*Serratia marcescens*
	Enterobacter species
Staphylococcus aureus	*Klebsiella pneumoniae*
Staphylococcus epidermidis	*Hemophilus influenzae* (uncommon in neonates)

loss of intact membranes allows direct access of vaginal bacteria to the fetus.

3. Maternal septicemia, transient bacteremia, or chorioamnionitis.
4. Birth asphyxia (hypoxia and acidosis may depress immune cellular functions).
5. Coitus occurring close to delivery carries an uncertain risk for maternal colonization and ultimately for fetal or neonatal infection.
6. Postnatal procedures such as intubation or catheterization of umbilical vessels increase the risk of infection.

SIGNS OF SEPSIS OR MENINGITIS IN NEONATES BY ORGAN SYSTEM

1. CNS: lethargy, early and persistent apnea (at less than 24 hr), fever (especially in meningitis) or temperature instability (greater than 1.5 C fluctuation) *or* warm trunk and cold extremities coexisting. Typical signs of meningitis in older children such as nuchal rigidity occur very late or never in the course of neonatal meningitis.
2. Respiratory: tachypnea, grunting, labored breathing, and apnea.
3. Gastrointestinal: feeding intolerance, especially vomiting, and large (>50%) gastric residuals of prior feedings, suggesting ileus.
4. Skin: gram-negative bacteria, especially Pseudomonas, may produce small necrotic lesions, especially on the face and trunk.
5. A directed physical examination should always include a search for signs of local infections such as scalp abscesses. Joint immobility or localized erythema (omphalitis) may also suggest localized manifestations of a generalized infection.

LABORATORY DATA

1. Leukopenia, especially neutropenia (less than 2000 total neutrophils and bands), extreme leukocytosis (more than 20,000 neutrophils and bands), or an increased (>0.2) ratio of immature neutrophils to mature forms may indicate sepsis.
2. Thrombocytopenia (less than 100,000 platelets/mm^3).
3. Metabolic acidosis.
4. Erythrocyte sedimentation rate (ESR) is not helpful as an isolated test.
5. Jaundice is not a reliable sign of bacterial sepsis in newborns.

No single clinical sign or single abnormal laboratory test is highly associated with sepsis, but combinations of the aforementioned signs strongly suggest sepsis or meningitis. Therefore, a prudent physician identifies infants at high risk and provides for extremely close observation of vital signs and overall status of those children during the first 24–48 hr of life.

DIAGNOSIS

1. Obtain blood culture (ideally 2 cultures from separate sites). The volume of blood should not be less than 10% of the culture medium volume.
2. Through a lumbar puncture, collect spinal fluid for at least a culture and a Gram's stain. Then perform a cell count and protein and glucose determinations. Pressure measurement is of little diagnostic use in newborns.
3. It may be wise to alert the clinical laboratory that only a small amount of spinal fluid will be available for analysis.
4. Urine obtained by suprapubic bladder aspiration is unlikely to demonstrate bacteria by culture or Gram's stain when obtained immediately after birth. An evaluation for sepsis performed several days after birth should, however, include an aspiration as a part of the diagnostic evaluation.

INITIAL STABILIZATION

General. Adequate warmth and correction of hypotension if observed (see chart p. 13) should be the first priorities. Central arterial pressure monitoring should be considered if such monitoring has not already been instituted.

The effects of vasopressor agents on neonates are relatively undocumented, but such agents may be indicated for hypotension and oliguria. We suggest dopamine 5–15 μg/kg/min infused into a secure intravenous site. Assisted ventilation may be necessary if apnea is severe or if sepsis is complicated by severe pneumonia.

Electrolyte imbalance almost always exists with meningitis, and a difficult therapeutic problem is balancing total fluid needs in a shocked infant with the need to correct the specific electrolyte abnormalities often present in meningitis.

Specific. Initial antibiotics for infections of undetermined etiology should be ampicillin and gentamicin. If a staphylococcal infection is strongly suspected, consider methicillin. If *Staphylococcus epidermidis* is recovered in culture and is resistant to methicillin, then consider vancomycin.

For enteric organisms resistant to ampicillin that are recovered from the spinal fluid, no single effective and safe antibiotic has gained great acceptance. Moxalactam, a newly developed antibiotic effective against many gram-negative organisms and able to penetrate into the cerebrospinal fluid (CFS), and chloramphenicol are both used in this situation. Aminoglycoside antibiotics have poor or variable CSF penetration and are therefore of limited usefulness in gram-negative meningitis. Intrathecal administration of aminoglycosides has been tested and shown not to be of value.

Correct coagulation abnormalities, which should be anticipated with significant sepsis of any bacterial etiology or with enteroviral infections. Platelet transfusions, or fresh frozen plasma or cryoprecipitate transfusions for correction of abnormal prothrombin or partial thromboplastin times, are indicated based on the specific abnormalities detected and the local availability of these products.

MANAGEMENT OF OVERWHELMING SEPSIS AND PNEUMONIA

The findings of overwhelming sepsis in neonates include respiratory failure, acidosis, extremely poor perfusion, hypotension, grunting respirations, evidence of hemorrhage (petechiae, purpura, pulmonary bleeding), neutropenia, and, eventually, sclerema.

There is now evidence that such afflicted infants lack specific opsonic antibodies in their pool of transplacentally acquired immunoglobulins. This limits the ability of the neutrophils to ingest and destroy bacteria. The extremely rapid growth of common infecting agents (Group B Streptococcus, *E. coli*) may create such a large total body burden of organisms that relative antibiotic resistance results.

Because of the extremely high mortality of such infants, several ancillary therapies have been tried in addition to the conventionally accepted treatments of assisted ventilation, crystalloid fluid administration, infusions of bicarbonate, antibiotics, and vasopressor agents. The first of these approaches consists of treatment to replace or supply specific immune factors. This may mean granulocyte transfusions in infants with neutropenia and total body depletion of neutrophils reflected in absent or decreased bone marrow stores, or infusion of pooled adult hyperimmune globulin to try to correct specific antibody deficiencies. The second approach is to correct these deficits and alter the oxygen-hemoglobin characteristics and oxygen tissue delivery characteristics of the infant's blood by complete exchange transfusion.

The efficacy of these treatments has not yet been proved; nor, given the difficulty of controlled clinical studies, is it likely to be proved soon. We favor replacement therapy with granulocyte transfusions, which provides large numbers of such cells without the added risks of exchange transfusion. Local blood bank practices may determine the optimal therapy for each locality. What is clear is that "immunotherapy" beyond conventional treatment may offer the only immediate hope for these unfortunate infants.

ADDITIONAL COMMENTS

1. A "healthy-appearing" neonate with bacteremia can become an infant in septic shock within a very few hours. An early sign of untreated (and too often of treated) sepsis is death.
2. The outcome of neonatal meningitis is related to the rapidity of clearance of organisms from the spinal fluid. Serial spinal punctures with assessment of culture findings, cell count, and perhaps antibiotic levels will help individualize therapy.
3. Infants evaluated for sepsis and initially treated far outnumber those with documented sepsis. Because of the vague nature of the signs and symptoms in neonates, the infant must remain under close observation for other conditions that may produce similar symptoms, such as hypoglycemia, electrolyte disturbances, or intracranial hemorrhage.
4. The duration of therapy for either sepsis or meningitis must be individualized based on the type of infectious agent, the briskness of clinical and (for meningitis), cellular response, and the likelihood of localized complications. For gram-negative enteric organisms or Group B streptococcal meningitis, at least 2 weeks' therapy following confirmed sterilization of the CSF is recommended, with further close follow-up thereafter.

Suggested management of infants at high risk for sepsis (e.g., born following prolonged rupture of membranes) is described in Table 14–2.

Gastric aspirate evaluations are not specific for indicating need for antibiotic treatment. An extremely abnormal white blood cell count or platelet count in an uncertain situation may support the suspicion of sepsis and prompt appropriate treatment. The more

Table 14–2. MANAGEMENT OF INFANT BORN FOLLOWING PROLONGED RUPTURE OF MEMBRANES, PROLONGED LABOR, OR MATERNAL FEVER

An infant born following prolonged rupture of membranes, prolonged labor, or maternal fever is at high risk for sepsis.

If asphyxiated or showing respiratory distress beyond 1 hr, evaluate and treat for sepsis.	If not asphyxiated and born at full term, then maintain close observation (incubator for 24 hr). If temperature fluctuates by more than 1.5 C in a stable incubator, if feedings are not tolerated, or if other signs develop during the first hours of life (cyanosis, apnea, lethargy), then evaluate and treat for sepsis.

premature the infant, the more likely a blood or spinal fluid culture will demonstrate the presence of sepsis or meningitis.

REFERENCES

1. Laurenti F, Ferro R, Isacchi G et al: Polymorphonuclear leukocyte transfusion for the treatment of sepsis in the newborn. J. Pediatr 98:118, 1981.
2. Lipuroky A, Palko J, Milner R, Akenzia G: The hematology of bacterial infections in premature infants. Pediatrics 57:839, 1976.
3. Pomerance J, Brand R, Meredith J: Differentiating environmental from disease-related fevers in the term newborn. Pediatrics 67:485, 1981.
4. Siegel J, McCracken G: Sepsis neonatorium. N Engl J Med 304:642, 1981.

LOCALIZED INFECTIONS THAT REPRESENT EMERGENCIES IN NEONATES

GONOCOCCAL NEONATAL OPHTHALMIA

An intense inflammatory reaction of the conjunctivae is produced by the localized growth of *Neisseria gonorrhoeae*. The lesions are found on the third to fifth day of life. Erythema and edema of the eyelids as well as a copious purulent discharge are present. Diagnosis is made by confirmation of the bacteria by culture and, more quickly, by Gram's stain examination, which reveals gram-negative diplococci and neutrophils. Other causes of conjunctivitis include chronic irritation, Chlamydia, and, rarely, Pseudomonas. Both Neisseria and Pseudomonas require specific therapy.

Therapy for gonococcal disease includes systemic penicillin

(50,000 U/kg/day q 8 hr) plus frequent saline irrigation of the eyes. Some also favor treatment with topical antibiotic drops (topical penicillin or chloramphenicol). Failure to control the infection may result in corneal ulceration and endophthalmitis. Silver nitrate drops may fail to prevent the disease when the drops are misplaced or washed out too rapidly. Therefore, an infant born to a woman with an endocervical culture positive for *N. gonorrhoeae* should receive one dose of penicillin (25,000 U intramuscularly) to provide more certain prophylaxis.

SEPTIC ARTHRITIS AND OSTEOMYELITIS

These conditions, which coexist in neonates because of a vascular link between the epiphyseal and metaphyseal circulatory systems, may present in neonates with typical signs of localized swelling, irritability, pain or palpation, decreased motion, or more subtle findings including edema of a distal extremity. Delay in diagnosis may result in permanent damage to the longitudinal growth potential of the bone. Diagnosis is made by aspiration of infected material from the joint space and concomitant growth of the offending organism (usually *Staphylococcus aureus,* even in neonates) from a blood culture.

Treatment is both orthopedic, with drainage of pus, and medical, with long term (4–6 week) continuation of antibiotic therapy. The specific antibiotic regimen will depend on the organism and the particular sensitivity pattern. *Candida albicans* and *N. gonorrhoeae* also produce this disease in neonates. A common location for osteomyelitis is the calcaneus, especially in prematures who are subjected to many heel punctures for blood drawing.

TOXIC EPIDERMAL NECROLYSIS

This occurs in newborns infected with certain strains of *S. aureus*. The disease produces large blistering areas that peel off with gentle rubbing, resulting in much fluid loss. Infants have many systemic signs of the illness. The principal differential diagnostic consideration is one of a variety of inherited blistering conditions that collectively are termed epidermolysis bullosa. Initial management of the staphylococcal infection consists of obtaining cultures of blood and cultures of the edges of the lesions, instituting antibiotic therapy with methicillin (100 mg/kg/day), and maintaining intravenous infusion for fluid replacement and, perhaps, protein replacement, as much protein may be lost from oozing of the open wounds. Infants are usually too ill initially to tolerate oral hydration. Prognosis is guarded.

DIARRHEA

In newborns diarrhea is usually not an emergency situation. Most cases are caused by *E. coli;* there is great potential for the rapid spread of this organism from infant to infant, and seriously ill infants may develop systemic disease. Strict attention to and treatment of fluid losses is the most critical part of therapy. Some treat with colistin or neomycin (12–25 mg/kg orally q 6 hr).

REFERENCES

1. Pittard W, Thullen J, Fanaroff A: Neonatal septic arthritis. J Pediatr 88:621, 1976.
2. Weissberg E, Smith A, Smith D: Clinical features of neonatal osteomyelitis. Pediatrics 53:505, 1974.

PRENATALLY ACQUIRED INFECTIOUS DISEASES

A variety of viral, spirochetal, and protozoal agents may infect the fetus, producing effects ranging from none, to first trimester abortion, to severe in utero disease with malformations and compromised postnatal life. Specific etiologic agents include spirochetes (*Treponema pallidum*), viruses (CMV, rubella, enterovirus), and protozoa (*Toxoplasma gondii*).

Because herpesvirus produces infections at delivery, it is considered in the following section of this chapter.

CLINICAL AND LABORATORY MANIFESTATIONS

1. Intrauterine growth retardation, especially of weight, but height and head circumference may also be affected.
2. Premature delivery.
3. Hepatomegaly and splenomegaly.
4. Hyperbilirubinemia, especially direct-reacting.
5. Skin lesions, especially purpura and petechiae.
6. Thrombocytopenia and disseminated intravascular coagulation.
7. Cerebral calcifications (most likely to be present at birth in toxoplasmosis).
8. Chorioretinitis (especially common in toxoplasmosis).
9. Periosteal elevation on long bone radiographic examination.
10. Hemolytic anemia.
11. Cataracts and congenital heart disease suggestive of congenital rubella.

DIAGNOSIS

1. Clinical suspicion of a viral infection and recovery of viral agents from nasopharyngeal, rectal, or urine cultures, or rising specific antibody titers during the first weeks of life, constitute firm diagnostic criteria.
2. For the diagnosis of syphilis, a positive Venereal Disease Research Laboratories (VDRL) test in the infant with a quantitative titer greater than that found in the mother, or rising or constant titers during the first weeks of life with a positive history in the mother, confirm the diagnosis.

TREATMENT

Syphilis

With CNS involvement (determined by clinical criteria or an abnormal spinal fluid), administer 50,000 U/kg q 24 hr × 21 days IM procaine penicillin or 50,000 U/kg/day q 12 hr × 14–21 days IV penicillin G. Without CNS involvement, administer 50,000 U/kg q 24 hr × 10 days IM procaine penicillin.

Toxoplasmosis

A possibly efficacious treatment consists of pyrimethamine 1 mg/kg/day q 12 hr and sulfadiazine 100–150 mg/kg/day q 6 hr × 30 days.

VIRAL ENTITIES

No specific antiviral agents have been proved effective to date with the exception of specific therapy for herpes simplex (see following section on herpes infections).

ADDITIONAL COMMENTS

1. The risk of exposure of nursery personnel to these agents is small, although some nurseries request that pregnant nursing personnel do not care for infants with any of the aforementioned infections.
2. Emergency aspects of management include resuscitation and investigation for a possibly treatable disease (syphilis) or minimization of further deficits likely to occur with infections for which no specific antimicrobial therapy is available. This last type of care consists of correction of thrombocytopenia and treatment of jaundice and hypoglycemia.

REFERENCES

1. Amstey M: Maternal viral infection with adverse results: cytomegalovirus and herpesvirus. Semin Perinatol 1:1, 1977.
2. Berry P, Nagington J: Fatal infection with echovirus II. Arch Dis Child 57:22, 1982.
3. Starr S: Cytomegalovirus. Pediatr Clin North Am 26:283, 1979.

HERPES SIMPLEX INFECTION OF THE NEWBORN

GENERAL CONSIDERATIONS

1. Herpes simplex virus (HSV) infection results from perinatal exposure to the virus because of clinically apparent or inapparent maternal genital infection. Seventy percent of mothers of HSV-infected infants are asymptomatic at delivery.
2. Because of the common nature of genital herpes infection in teenagers, there is a high risk of exposure and infection in infants born to teenage mothers.
3. Cesarean section is indicated if the mother has signs of active infection or if she has virologic culture evidence of herpes and the membranes are ruptured for less than 4–6 hr. Beyond this time fetal exposure will have already occurred, and there is no advantage to the fetus in performing a cesarean section.
4. This infection is considered separately from other viral infections because it does not typically occur in utero and because clinical outcome in the neonate can be modified by antiviral agents.

PRESENTATION

1. Prenatal infection is rare. HSV-infected infants do not demonstrate the same types of lesions that other viruses (including other DNA viruses such as CMV) demonstrate at birth. However, 50% of infants who develop HSV infections are delivered after less than 38 weeks' gestation, and a disproportionate number appear to have complicated neonatal courses prior to the clinical onset of the disease.
2. The mean age of presentation is 16 days, but the range can be from 1 day to 6 weeks.
3. Three clinical patterns of onset have been recognized:
   a. Isolated CNS disease with symptoms of lethargy, poor feeding, and an unstable core temperature. CSF examination reveals pleocytosis and elevated protein concentration.
   b. Isolated skin and eye disease. Infants develop a single skin

vesicle or clusters of vesicles 1 mm to 1 cm in diameter on a mildly erythematous base, most commonly occurring over presenting parts such as the skin of the face, the scalp, the eyes, or mucous membranes, especially of the mouth. Lesions are variable in appearance but are most often vesicular.

c. Disseminated disease presents in infants with signs of liver dysfunction (elevated SGOT and SGPT levels, jaundice, and hepatomegaly), pneumonia, and coagulopathy. They may also have CNS disease, often manifested as seizures.

All infants with herpes have a potentially lethal disease. Seventy percent of the infants with cutaneous manifestations only will develop disseminated disease during their course. Twenty percent of newborns with HSV never have skin involvement, although 70% of infants with HSV present with skin lesions alone.

DIAGNOSIS

Diagnosis is confirmed by isolation of the virus from the skin, urine, stools, CSF, or brain biopsy tissue. Cultures may require 72 hr or more to demonstrate growth. A diagnosis can be made more rapidly with a direct immunofluorescence technique available only in certain hospitals.

MANAGEMENT

1. Because of the overwhelming mortality and morbidity of the disease and the new possibility of specific treatment, the physician must act promptly in any suspected case of HSV:
   a. Obtain cultures of likely sites of viral growth.
   b. Obtain immunofluorescent studies of skin lesions.
   c. Isolate the infant.
   d. Isolate the mother if she is still hospitalized. Teach her that she must wash her hands carefully and refrain from kissing the baby if she has a herpetic cold sore.
   e. A culture of the mother's cervix up to 3 weeks' post partum may still reveal the virus.
   f. Transfer the infant to a center where antiviral therapy is possible.
2. General care is supportive in nature with special efforts to prevent hypothermia, which may enhance dissemination.
3. Two agents are possibly effective as antiviral therapy: vidarabine (adenosine arabinoside) and acycloguanine (acyclovir). Either should be administered as soon as the diagnosis can be confirmed. When tested against a placebo, vidarabine (10–20 mg/kg/day for 2 weeks) decreased mortality in severe disease

and may have decreased overall morbidity. At present, a clinical trial comparing the two agents in neonatal HSV infection is under way.

ADDITIONAL COMMENTS

1. Without skin or eye lesions from which culture material can be easily obtained, the infant with herpes infection limited to the CNS is extremely difficult to diagnose, as other infectious and noninfectious causes of systemic and especially CNS disease in the newborn may have a similar clinical appearance. Cultures of material from either parent may be of some help and are clearly less invasive than brain biopsy of the infant. However, brain biopsy may sometimes be required to make the diagnosis. Localizing EEG findings may guide the use of brain biopsy.
2. Although children with skin lesions alone are likely to survive, some of them may have later neurointellectual deficits because of a clinically inapparent extension of the disease to the nervous system.

REFERENCES

1. Brunell P: Prevention and treatment of neonatal herpes. Pediatrics 66:806, 1980.
2. Committee of the Fetus and Newborn: Perinatal herpes simplex virus infection. Pediatrics 66:147, 1980.
3. Whitely R, Nahmias A, Vinistine A et al: The natural history of herpes simplex virus infection of mother and newborn. Pediatrics 66:489, 1980.

15

NEUROLOGIC DISORDERS

SEIZURES

GENERAL CONSIDERATIONS

1. Seizures are a frequent and serious problem in a NICU. The frequency among premature infants requiring intensive care is about 20–25%.
2. The overall frequency is about 1/1000 live births.
3. The presence of seizures is an important predictor of subsequent neurologic impairment when not caused by hypoglycemia or hypocalcemia.
4. Treatment is often frustrating, as seizures are difficult to control for first day or two with drugs available at present.
5. Since seizures may interfere with respiration, it is important to recognize their presence, to discover their underlying causes, and to minimize their damage.
6. Seizures are often difficult to recognize, particularly in the premature infant, as signs may be subtle.
7. Although there are many possible etiologies, asphyxia is the most common cause.

ETIOLOGY

1. Asphyxia.
2. Intracranial hemorrhage:
   a. Subependymal, intraventricular, cortical.
   b. Birth trauma (subarachnoid, subdural, cortical contusion).
   c. A-V malformation.
   d. Thrombocytopenia.
   e. Hemorrhagic disease of the newborn.
   f. Cortical vein thrombosis.
3. Metabolic:
   a. Hypoglycemia.
   b. Hypocalcemia.
   c. Hypernatremia.
   d. Hyponatremia.
   e. Hypomagnesemia.
   f. Hyperammonemia.
4. Infection:
   a. Meningitis (bacterial).
   b. Viral meningoencephalitis (herpes, CMV, coxsackie, rubella).

   c. Toxoplasmosis.
   d. Syphilis.
5. Withdrawal from passive addiction to maternal drugs (see Chapter 2).
6. Chromosomal anomalies (4p minus, trisomy 13 or 18).
7. Genetic disorders:
   a. Congenital lactic acidosis.
   b. Phakomatoses.
   c. Cerebrohepatorenal syndrome.
   d. Smith-Lemli-Opitz syndrome.
8. Amino acid disorders:
   a. Urea cycle defects (carbamyl phosphate synthetase, ornithine transcarbamylase, argininosuccinic acid synthetase).
   b. Nonketotic hyperglycinemia (glycine decarboxylase).
   c. Hyperlysinemia.
   d. Maple syrup urine disease (leucine, isoleucine, valine).
   e. Hyperbeta-alaninemia.
   f. Sarcosinemia.
   g. Carnosinemia.
   h. Phenylketonuria.
   i. Hyperornithinemia, homocitrullinemia.
9. Organic acid disorders (metabolic acidosis):
   a. Propionic acidemia.
   b. Methylmalonic acidemia.
   c. Beta-ketothiolase.
   d. Pyruvate dehydrogenase, pyruvate carboxylase deficiency.
   e. Fructose 1–6 diphosphatase deficiency.
   f. Glycogen storage disease type I.
   g. Maple syrup urine disease.
   h. Isovaleric acidemia.
10. Congenital malformations:
   a. Lissencephaly.
   b. Porencephaly.
   c. Polymicrogyria.
11. Miscellaneous:
   a. Pyridoxine dependency
   b. Galactosemia.
   c. Gaucher's disease.
   d. Polycythemia.
   e. Intravenous injection of local anesthetic.
   f. Kernicterus.

PRESENTATION

1. Clinical manifestations differ among premature and full term infants.
2. Accompanying signs of asphyxia are often present.

3. Frank seizures may be tonic, clonic, general, localized, fragmentary, asynchronous, or asymmetric.
4. Subtle manifestations, particularly in premature infants, include tonic extensor tone, apnea (often without major changes in heart rate), irritability, and jitteriness.
5. Less subtle signs include bicycling movement of the lower extremities, flailing of arms, blinking, staring, tonic deviation of the eyes, sucking, mouthing, and repetitive motions.
6. Sustained tonic activity should rouse suspicions of structural brain disease.
7. Localized or focal seizure activity is not necessarily indicative of focal disease.
8. Some seizures will be manifested by prolonged apnea and cyanosis.

DIAGNOSIS

Clinical

1. When considering the preceding list of etiologies, note any history of possible asphyxia (prenatal, intrapartum, or postnatal) and the family history.
2. A premature infant < 1500 g birth weight is at risk for intraventricular hemorrhage (IVH).
3. Transillumination of skull.
4. Bulging or tense fontanel.

Laboratory

1. Blood: glucose, Ca^{++}, Mg^{++}, pH, PaO_2, $PaCO_2$, serum electrolytes, and ammonia.
2. Urine: amino acids, galactose, and toxic screen.
3. Lumbar puncture: white blood count (WBC), red blood count (RBC), and cultures.
4. VDRL test, culture or serologic evidence of viral infection.

CT Scan. Anomalies, infarction, hemorrhage, displacement, or calcifications.

EEG

1. Variable patterns.
2. Paroxysmal discharges, repetitive spike, rhythmic delta activity, and sometimes minimal changes. Signs in prematures of less than 32 weeks' gestational age are more subtle than those in full term infants.
3. Has prognostic significance if abnormal during the first few days of life.
4. Abnormal patterns of EEG activity often become normal at several days of age.

Ultrasonography

1. IVH in premature.
2. Deviated midline structure.
3. Malformations.

Skull Radiograph. Rarely helpful or indicated.

TREATMENT

1. If hypoglycemic: administer IV D10–15W 4–5 mL/kg, then D10W 8–10 mg/kg/min with frequent rechecks to assess adequacy of treatment.
   If normoglycemic: administer IV D10W 80 mL/kg/day.
2. If hypocalcemic: administer IV 10% calcium gluconate 2 mL/kg.
3. If hypomagnesemic: administer IM 50% $MgSO_4$ 0.2 mL/kg.
4. Phenobarbital: IV loading dose is 20 mg/kg (2 doses of 10 mg/kg over 5–10 min). Maintain at 5–10 mg/kg/day (2 oral or IV doses), then decrease to 3–4 mg/kg/day. Serum level should be 20–30 mcg/mL.
5. Phenytoin: add if phenobarbital is unsuccessful over 4–6 hr, depending on the frequency and severity of seizures. The IV loading dose is 10–15 mg/kg, IV maintenance dose is 2–4 mg/kg, and the serum level should be 15–20 mcg/mL. Oral and IM routes are not satisfactory.
6. Paraldehyde: if there is no response from phenobarbital or phenytoin, administer an IV or IM dose of 0.3 mL/kg rectally (most common route).
7. Diazepam: this drug is rarely used. It is short-acting and causes vasodilation and hypotension. Administer (slowly) a variable IV dose of 0.1–0.3 mg/kg.
8. Pyridoxine: if seizures do not respond to anticonvulsant medication, administer 50 mg intravenously, with one trial during a seizure.

Long Term. Usually continue phenobarbital (sometimes phenytoin also) at least through the first 6 months of life.

ADDITIONAL COMMENTS

The long term prognosis will depend on the etiology, severity, and duration of the seizures. Prolonged seizures generally have a poor neurologic outcome. Seizures that are of short duration and few in number (3 or 4) have a much better outlook. The presence of other neurologic signs at time of discharge (e.g., floppiness, poor feeding, poor tone) heralds a poor outcome.

REFERENCES

1. Baska RE: Seizure Disorders. *In* Coleman M (ed): Neonatal Neurology. Baltimore, University Press, 1981, p. 177.
2. Bergman I, Painter MJ, Crumrine PK: Neonatal seizures. Semin Perinatol 6:54, 1982.
3. Neonatal Seizures. *In* Volpe JJ (ed): Neurology of the Newborn. Philadelphia, Saunders, 1981, p. 111.

INTRACRANIAL HEMORRHAGES

SUBEPENDYMAL HEMORRHAGE

General Considerations

Subependymal hemorrhage (SEH) occurs in 40–50% of premature infants weighing less than 1500 g at birth. The common site of bleeding is the germinal matrix at the level of the caudate nucleus or the thalamus. This area is rich in blood vessels and poor in supporting parenchymal tissue. Extravasated blood often breaks through the adjacent ependyma into the ventricle and may extend further into the brain tissue.

Classification

Grade I. Confined to subependymal area.

Grade II. Subependymal and intraventricular blood without ventricular dilation.

Grade III. Subependymal and intraventricular blood with ventricular dilation.

Grade IV. Subependymal, intraventricular blood, ventricular dilation, and extension of blood into brain parenchyma.

Blood will often extend from the choroid plexus through the foramen of Monro to the third ventricle.

The cause is unknown, but several etiologic factors have been suggested, including a rich developing capillary network; poor supporting structures; hypoxia; venous congestion; hypotension; hypertension; changes in cerebral blood flow secondary to pH, PaO_2, or $PaCO_2$; lack of autoregulation of cerebral blood flow; endothelial injury; increased blood volume (plasma volume expansion); hyperosmolarity ($NaHCO_3$ infusion); and abnormalities in coagulation factors.

Presentation

Clinical indications include difficult delivery, low Apgar score, perinatal asphyxia, and less than 32 weeks' gestation. Hemorrhages may also occur in more mature infants.

Rapid clinical deterioration may occur together with a condition resembling shock, loss of neuromuscular tone, seizures, and apnea. However, significant hemorrhage can occur without apparent signs, and therefore the timing of the hemorrhage is difficult to determine. Most occur during the first 72 hr after birth, but some are delayed till the second week of life. Clinical signs may be insidious or dramatic, with marked obtundation of the infant or no changes apart from a fall in the hematocrit level. There may be a subtle or slow deterioration with less activity, increasing apneic episodes, bradycardia, and hypotonia.

Diagnosis

History. As above—perinatal asphyxia.

Clinical. Variable and unreliable.

Laboratory. CSF is often bloody with high protein. LP is generally not helpful.

Sonar Scan. Most useful in detecting site and extent. Repeat at weekly intervals until the patient is stabilized.

CT Scan. Helps to delineate ventricular size or other sites of parenchymal damage. It is indicated if signs appear after the first week.

Therapy

Grades I–II. Observation.

Grades III–IV. There is some question as to whether hydrocephalus can be prevented. Some have advocated daily LPs to prevent pressure build-up, but this treatment has not been verified by appropriately controlled studies. The incidence of hydrocephalus appears to be less than 10%. If occipital-frontal circumference (OFC) continues to increase out of proportion to body growth and there is increasing ventricular dilatation, then a ventriculoperitoneal shunt is indicated.

Additional Comments

Further studies are needed to determine the long term neurologic sequelae, especially of Grades I and II hemorrhages, which warrant initial optimism. It is unclear whether the hemorrhage itself or its cause (e.g., hypoxia) is more important in producing permanent damage. The mortality rate is high among infants with Grade IV hemorrhage, and therefore extensive follow-up information on these infants is not available.

SUBARACHNOID HEMORRHAGE

General Considerations

Hemorrhage within the subarachnoid space (SAH) can occur as a primary lesion or secondary to intracerebral hemorrhage. Whereas IVH is common, a significant SAH is uncommon in the premature infant. Small amounts of blood in the subarachnoid space are probably common and inconsequential in both term and preterm infants. A primary hemorrhage results from tears of bridging veins within the subarachnoid space or of small leptomeningeal vessels, which are usually more marked over the cerebral convexities. Major or secondary hemorrhage may occur in association with an IVH, vascular malformations (vein of Galen aneurysm, A–V fistula), or severe coagulopathy.

Presentation

1. Minor bleeding is most common, especially in premature infants. There are minimal or no signs.
2. Moderate bleeding occurs more often in full term infants and may be associated with prolonged or difficult delivery. Seizures may occur on second day of life in an otherwise asymptomatic infant.
3. Massive hemorrhage usually occurs in a critically ill infant with other neurologic signs—severe asphyxia or trauma at birth, seizures, shock, or coma. It is often fatal and may be associated with structural CNS anomalies.

Diagnosis

History. Asphyxia or trauma at delivery.

Clinical. Varies from asymptomatic to marked CNS abnormalities, including seizures.

Lumbar Puncture. Spinal fluid may be grossly bloody or contain only microscopic evidence of blood. Protein is elevated.

CT Scan. This may reveal abnormal density over cerebral convexities.

Sonar Scan. This will rule out SEH and IVH but will not detect SAH.

Therapy

Therapy should be conservative. Observe for hydrocephalus.

Additional Comments

The prognosis of infants with SAH, including those with seizures, is generally good; however, associated CNS lesions will determine neurologic sequelae. The major complication is hydrocephalus secondary to altered CSF absorption or obstruction to CSF flow.

SUBDURAL HEMATOMA

General Considerations

Subdural hematomas have become rare with modern day obstetric practice. Small hematomas may occur in the posterior or middle fossa and are almost always secondary to trauma. The source of the bleeding may be the small pial veins joining the longitudinal sinus adjacent to overriding suture lines or the tearing of tributaries of the vein of Galen. Hematomas occur more commonly in full term than in premature infants.

Presentation

Hemorrhage Over Cortex (Convexity Hematoma). This is more common in full term than in preterm infants and results from tearing of the bridging veins during compression and molding of the head at birth. It occurs more frequently over the frontoparietal region but can occur over the entire cortex.

The signs vary from minimal to marked, and onset may be delayed 1 to several days. Signs include irritability, pallor, seizures (usually focal), bulging fontanel, retinal hemorrhages, hemiparesis, deviation of eyes toward the hemiparetic side, intact doll's eye reflex, and anisocoria. There often is little correlation between the extent of the hemorrhage and the severity of clinical findings.

Convexity hematomas are most often associated with a cerebral contusion, and the resulting signs will predominate.

Posterior Fossa Hemorrhage (Falcial and Tentorial Tears). These are more common in full term infants. They generally occur with a tentorial or falcial laceration during a difficult or traumatic delivery and involve adjacent vessels: the vein of Galen, the lateral sinus, the straight sinus, or the inferior sagital sinus. The onset of signs is usually immediate, but it can be delayed. Signs may include irritability, a high-pitched cry, lethargy, hypotonia, stupor, and nuchal rigidity.

If a hemorrhage enlarges or compresses the fourth ventricle, intracranial pressure will increase or brain stem compression will occur with anisocoria, nystagmus, or fixed dilated pupils progressing to respiratory arrest.

Diagnosis

History. Inquire about prolonged labor, cephalopelvic disproportion, difficult delivery, or birth trauma.

Clinical. Signs are variable, as above. Distinguish between convexity and posterior fossa hematoma with brain stem signs.

Transillumination. Fresh blood will *decrease* the amount of light transmitted compared with the normal side. This technique is not helpful if the hemorrhage is diffuse or if scalp hemorrhage has occurred.

Skull Radiographs. These are generally not helpful since fractures are not usually associated. If occipital osteodiastasis is suspected, a lateral skull film will reveal the inward protrusion of the occipital bone.

CT Scan. This will reveal a rim-like collection of blood with convexity hematoma, a midline density (linear or circular) with a falcial hemorrhage, and a density in the posterior fossa with a tentorial tear. A large hematoma will cause a shift of midline structures.

Ultrasonography. This will not detect convexity hematoma, but it may detect posterior fossa hemorrhage, and it will detect a midline shift.

Subdural Taps. These are definitive. Use a No. 22 gauge short bevel spinal needle with obturator.

Therapy

Convexity Hematoma. Subdural taps can relieve pressure but should not be repeated if the infant is asymptomatic and OFC is not increasing (see Chapter 20, Emergency Procedures).

Tentorial or Falcial Tears. There is no practical treatment. The immediate outlook is poor. Surgical evacuation is possible if it is performed rapidly.

Additional Comments

A subdural hematoma may occur at the time of birth and present few if any signs during the neonatal period. A chronic subdural effusion can develop over several months, presenting with an enlarged head, increased transillumination, and a bulging fontanel.

CEREBELLAR HEMORRHAGE

General Considerations

Isolated hemorrhage into the cerebellum is rare; however, in an infant of less than 1500 g with a marked IVH, bleeding may extend into the cerebellum. Other sources of hemorrhage include rupture of small subpial vessels, tear of the occipital sinus, laceration of the cerebellum (occipital diastasis), and venous thrombosis.

The pathogenesis is unclear, although there is a strong association with IVH, hypoxia, and severe prematurity. Obstruction of the venous sinuses by external compression during delivery or prolonged application of a face mask for mechanical ventilation has been implicated. Increases in blood pressure or blood flow may rupture capillaries in the cerebellar germinal matrix in SEH.

Presentation

There is generally a history of asphyxia, and the infant is most commonly premature and suffering from hyaline membrane disease. Sudden severe apnea associated with bradycardia may occur, usually after the second day of life. There may also be a sudden deterioration with hypotension and low hematocrit levels.

Diagnosis

CT Scan. Measure density in posterior fossa.

Cranial Ultrasonography. This is less reliable than a CT scan, but it may detect posterior fossa density.

Bloody CSF. LP is not indicated if cerebellar hemorrhage is suspected because of the possible risk of herniating the cerebellum through the foramen magnum.

Therapy

1. Treat cardiovascular and respiratory instability.
2. Observe for hydrocephalus.

3. Successful surgical evacuation of cerebellar hematoma has been reported.

REFERENCES

1. Abrams IF, McLennan JE, Mandell F: Acute neonatal subdural hematoma following breech delivery. Am J Dis Child 131:192, 1977.
2. Blank NK, Strand R, Gilles FH et al: Posterior fossa subdural hematomas in neonates. Arch Neurol 35:108, 1978.
3. Lebed MR, Schafrim BS, Waffran F et al: Real-time B scanning in the diagnosis of neonatal intracranial hemorrhage. Am J Obstet Gynecol 142:851, 1982.
4. Mack LA, Wright K, Hirsch JH et al: Intracranial hemorrhage in premature infants: accuracy of sonographic evaluation. AJR 137:245, 1981.
5. Shinnar S, Molteni RA, Gammon K et al: Intraventricular hemorrhage in the premature infant. A changing outlook. N Engl J Med 306:1464, 1982.
6. Volpe JJ: Neonatal intraventricular hemorrhage. N Engl J Med 304:886, 1981.
7. Volpe JJ: Neurology of the Newborn. Philadelphia, Saunders, 1981, p. 239.
8. Wigglesworth JS, Pape KE: Pathophysiology of intracranial hemorrhage in the newborn. J Perinat Med 8:119, 1980.

MALFORMATIONS OF THE CENTRAL NERVOUS SYSTEM

GENERAL CONSIDERATIONS

Malformations involving the central nervous system are relatively common and second in overall incidence only to congenital heart disease. Approximately one third of all recognizable malformations in the newborn involve the central nervous system, with an incidence of 0.5–1.5/1000 live births. The most common problems are those that involve defects of the neural groove and its failure to close, resulting in anencephaly or meningomyelocele. Some defects have a genetic predisposition and others are chromosomal, but the vast majority are unexplained. It is difficult to identify teratogens or determine the precise time of injury during embryonic development. The widespread use of ultrasonography for screening and the determination of alpha-fetoprotein in amniotic fluid have permitted the diagnosis of a number of central nervous system malformations prior to birth.

PRESENTATION

Anomalies of the First and Dorsal Phases of Neural Tube Formation

These anomalies, including anencephaly, occur between 17 and 30 days of embryonic life.

Anencephaly. Incidence ranges from 1/250 (Ireland) to 1/2500 births (Soviet Union). The infant has a frog-like appearance, with the crown of the head flattened, the eyes bulging, a plump nose, and a large or protruding tongue. The frontal bones are absent. The remainder of the body is normal, although there may be overgrowth of the upper extremities. The optic chiasm is present, the forebrain is absent, and the brain defect may be more extensive, involving the base of the brain. The pituitary is usually present and the hypothalamus absent. There is adrenal hypoplasia. The chance of a second sibling's having anencephaly is 6.8%; with two previous siblings, the chance of a third infant is increased to 56%.

Iniencephaly. This is anencephaly with an extreme retroflexion of the spine so that the face looks upward. It is often fatal prior to birth.

Klippel-Feil Syndrome. This is a more minor defect that is quite compatible with life. It is characterized by fusion of part or all the cervical spine with a reduced or normal number of cervical vertebrae. The CNS is usually intact, but there may be anomalies of the occipital bone. The neck is usually short, with a low hairline. There are three categories: (1) massive fusion of the cervical vertebrae, (2) fusions at one or more interspaces of the cervical vertebrae, and (3) fusions of cervical and lower thoracic or lumbar vertebrae. These fusions have been described in fetal alcohol syndrome.

Exencephaly. This is a severe anomaly with the brain developed entirely outside of the skull. The neural tube degenerates as the fetus matures in the uterus, and there is no skull formation.

Myeloschisis. The spinal cord is flat, plate-like, and covered by connective tissue. The spinal column fails to fuse with absent spinal processes, and the spinal root ganglia are aberrant. The infant usually does not survive the first week of life.

Spina Bifida Occulta. This is a very common lesion of spinal dysraphism affecting 10–20% of the population. The lesion most commonly affects vertebrae L5 and S1, although it can occur anywhere in the spinal column. It is not considered a pathologic finding if there are no signs or symptoms.

Meningomyelocele. This is the most common malformation of the CNS occurring in the neonatal period. The lesion is evident as a skin defect over the lower back, usually covered by a membrane. Because of spinal fluid accumulation under this membrane, a bulge forms. Most infants with meningomyelocele also have a structural abnormality of the brain stem and cerebellum: the Arnold-Chiari malformation. Because of this defect, hydrocephalus will commonly develop in the first days after birth. Functional defects with meningomyelocele may include denervated, flaccid lower extremities, congenital hip dislocations, foot deformities, absent anal reflex, and urinary dribbling because of defective bladder innervation. Additionally, these infants must be watched for signs of cranial nerve dysfunction, such as absent or depressed gag reflex, stridulous respirations, and apneic and bradycardic spells.

After recognizing the lesion, the physician should cover the defect with sterile saline-soaked gauze and keep the infant on a sterile towel until definitive surgical closure of the defect is performed. This is best done in a multidisciplinary setting. Any transfer of such an infant requires heart rate monitoring because of the risk of apnea and bradycardia.

Prognosis depends on the location of the lesion and the associated defects.

Anomalies of the Second and Third Phases of Neural Tube Formation

Following the closure of the neural tube, the lower lumbar, sacral, and coccygeal segments develop from stages 13 through 20 of embryonic life. Neural differentiation occurring in the tail fold consists of enlarging vacuoles that make contact with the central canal, a process called canalization.

Diastematomyelia. The spinal cord splits longitudinally into two discrete portions. This malformation is often associated with a bony spicula or fibrous band arising from the vertebral body, with other severe defects such as anencephaly or myelomeningocele, or with signs of cutaneous, bladder, or neuromuscular abnormalities. The most common sites are vertebrae L3, L4, and T10. It is unusual to diagnose this condition in the immediate newborn period. Treatment consists of surgery.

Meningocele. Incidence is 1/10,000 live births. The posterior spinal process fails to fuse, resulting in a dorsal prolapse of arachnoid and dura mater. The spinal cord is intact, and there are no neurologic deficits. Therefore, surgical repair is elective and in part cosmetic. Usually meningocele is not associated with other anomalies.

Lipomas. The formation of a lumbosacral lipoma can compress the spinal cord. It is sometimes associated with meningocele and may occur without signs. Most often it is not diagnosed in the neonatal period.

Myelocystocele. This is a cystic mass over the lower spinal area covered with skin and glia. It is associated with cloacal exstrophy and other malformations, including agenesis of the sacral vertebrae with motor and sensory deficits of the lower extremities.

Holoprosencephaly. This lesion occurs when diverticulation or cleavage of the olfactory, optic, or telencephalic vesicles is disrupted or arrested. The embryonic prosencephalon is retained to varying degrees, ranging from an undivided cerebrum with a single ventricle to minor anomalies such as dysplasia of the olfactory bulbs. The defect is also known as arhinencephaly or holotelencephaly. There are three major types—alobar, semilobar, and lobar—representing a spectrum of disorders in which there is a failure of midline cleavage of the forebrain and therefore a wide variation in neurologic outcome. Dysmorphic facies are common and may include cyclops, absence of nose, misplaced nose above the eye, absent facial bones, ocular hypotelorism, flat nose, median cleft lip, ethmocephaly, cebocephaly, and premaxillary agenesis. Holoprosencephaly occurs in association with chromosomal defects trisomy 13 and 13q, ring 13, and trisomy 18 and 18P.

Anomalies of the Cortex

Lissencephaly. This results in microcephaly, a high forehead, a prominent occiput, micrognathia, hirsutism, and an incomplete helix (ears). Associated defects include polydactyly, omphalocele, heart and kidney anomalies, micromelia, club feet, and opisthotonos.

Pachygyria. Gyri are wide and few in number. The defect is associated with wide and shallow sulci, spasticity, seizures, and opisthotonos.

Polymicrogyria. Gyri are small and increased in number. The defect is associated with seizures and cerebrohepatorenal syndrome.

Ulegyria. This involves cortical nodular sclerosis—atrophy of limited portions of the brain, particularly the frontal or parieto-occipital cortex (''walnut brain''). It is associated with seizures and with other congenital lesions.

Schizencephaly. There is a cleft-like defect in cortex involving absence of the corpus callosum, hydrocephalus, and an absent septum pellucidum. Marked CNS signs include lethargy, hypotonia, seizures, decerebrate posturing, and opisthotonos.

Hydranencephaly. The part of the brain perfused by carotid arteries is absent. There is marked transillumination of the skull.

The infant may appear normal at birth. Duration of survival depends on the presence of the hypothalamus.

Agenesis of Corpus Callosum. There may be complete separation of the hemispheres. Usually, there are no neurologic signs in newborns. It is discovered by CT scan or ultrasonography.

Encephalocele. A cranial defect resulting in protrusion of brain "within" the meninges (meningoencephalocele, encephalocystocele, hydranencephalocele), mostly in the occipital regions. Survival is approximately 50%. With just a meningocele, the prognosis is very good.

Porencephaly. A cavity within the brain communicating with the ventricles can result from infection, ischemia, trauma, or hemorrhage. It is associated with CMV and follows Grade IV intracranial hemorrhage. Variable neurologic signs depend on the size and location.

REFERENCES

1. Lemire RJ, Loeser JD, Leech RW et al: Normal and Abnormal Development of the Human Nervous System. Hagerstown, Md., Harper & Row, 1975.
2. Warkany J: Congenital Malformations. Chicago, Year Book, 1971.

CRANIAL TRAUMA

GENERAL CONSIDERATIONS

Most deliveries are probably accompanied by some trauma to the head. Fortunately, with modern day obstetrics significant injury to the CNS is rare. The most common forms of cranial trauma are exterior to the brain and include caput succedaneum, subgaleal hemorrhage, and cephalhematoma. Skull fractures are rare thanks to decreased use of forceps extraction in vaginal deliveries and more common use of cesarean sections for cephalopelvic disproportion. (See also Chapter 3, section on Birth Injuries.)

Caput Succedaneum. Soft tissue swelling characterized by pitting hemorrhagic edema over the vertex is extremely common following vertex vaginal deliveries. The swelling is a result of pressure on the subcutaneous tissues and is usually accompanied by marked molding of the head. The cap-like swelling generally crosses cranial suture lines.
Treatment. None. The condition usually resolves over several days.

Cephalhematoma. This subperiosteal hematoma occurs in 1–2% of all infants and is commonly associated with primiparas and forceps-assisted deliveries. About one third of mid-forceps deliveries result in a hematoma. The lesion presents as circumscribed, hard, and often unilateral swelling over a cranial bone, usually the parietal bone. It develops several hours or days after birth and is often accompanied by an underlying skull fracture. The hematoma generally increases after birth, the margins becoming firm and elevated, with a depressed center mimicking a depressed skull fracture. It does not transilluminate.

Treatment. None. The swelling decreases gradually, usually subsiding in 1 to 3 weeks. If calcification occurs, the hematoma may last for months. Increased breakdown of red blood cells within the closed space may contribute to jaundice. Needle aspiration is contraindicated owing to the risk of infection.

Subgaleal Hematoma. This type of injury is relatively rare and results from hemorrhage beneath the epicranial aponeurosis. The bleeding may be extensive, spreading beneath the entire scalp and over the neck. The major concern is blood loss; therefore, it is important to recognize the swelling as blood-containing.

Skull Fractures. These may be linear or depressed and most commonly involve the parietal bone. A linear fracture is often difficult to detect unless there are other signs of CNS injury, such as intracranial hemorrhage or a cephalhematoma. A depressed skull fracture may present as an inward depression or a "ping-pong" indentation and is almost always the result of a difficult vaginal delivery and the use of forceps. A bony defect is palpable with the depression, and a skull radiograph provides confirmation. Other CNS signs are rare.

Treatment. None for a linear fracture. A CT scan should be done to determine the presence of intracranial hemorrhage. The treatment for a depressed fracture is controversial. Some lesions will spontaneously elevate, and there are reports of successful elevation by suction with a breast pump or an obstetric vacuum extractor. A CT scan is indicated to rule out extradural or subdural hemorrhage followed by close observation. Surgical elevation is indicated in the presence of focal neurologic signs. The ping-pong lesions do not require treatment.

16

HEMATOLOGIC DISORDERS

POLYCYTHEMIA

GENERAL CONSIDERATIONS

1. Polycythemia, an absolute increase in the circulating red cell mass, predisposes to hyperviscosity (sludging) of the flow of cells and fluid in small vessels and capillaries. Not all polycythemic infants are hyperviscous, but virtually all hyperviscous infants are polycythemic.
2. The newborn has a normal hematocrit range of 50–60%, which is relatively polycythemic by normal adult standards. This increased erythrocyte mass presumably results from chronic in utero hypoxic stimulation of the manufacture and release of new erythrocytes.

INFANTS AT RISK FOR DEVELOPING POLYCYTHEMIA

1. Infants with delayed clamping of the umbilical cord (home deliveries, uncontrolled deliveries, "fad" deliveries).
2. Infants with evidence of marginal placental function (SGA infants).
3. Infants with active erythropoiesis secondary to fetal insulin stimulation (IDF or unexplained LGA infants).
4. A certain percentage of term infants without detectable predisposing conditions will also be polycythemic.

CLINICAL FINDINGS

Clinical findings tend to be absent or very obscure. Among those reported and referable to the CNS are apnea, jitteriness, fluctuating levels of consciousness, lethargy, and hypotonia. There may also be cyanotic episodes or unexplained color changes.

Laboratory Findings

1. Chest radiography may show cardiomegaly with increased peripheral vascular markings and perhaps evidence of pleural or parenchymal fluid.
2. Associated abnormalities include hypoglycemia and thrombocytopenia.

DIAGNOSIS

1. A venipuncture (not heel stick) hematocrit level is the appropriate diagnostic test, although a heel stick level may be useful for screening purposes. Warmed heel puncture hematocrit determinations will be 5–15% greater than simultaneously obtained venipuncture hematocrit levels when both are obtained during the first 2–24 hr of life. Venipuncture hematocrit determinations of higher than 65% and especially higher than 70% are associated with hyperviscosity and usually with clinical symptoms.
2. A viscometer allows for more direct measurement of the hyperviscous state but is not yet in widespread clinical use.

TREATMENT

1. Correction of the most emergent metabolic abnormality is achieved by IV or oral administration of glucose-containing fluids.
2. Careful temperature control is important. Overheating and subsequent increased free water loss are to be avoided, or a more critical hematocrit elevation may occur.
3. Partial exchange transfusion to lower the hematocrit level is indicated. Acceptable replacement fluids include physiologic saline, Ringer's lactate solution, fresh frozen plasma, or 5% albumin mixed with saline.
4. Exchange volume is calculated by the following formula:
$$\text{Ex Vol} = \frac{(\text{BV} \times [\text{Obs. Hct} - \text{Desired Hct}])}{\text{Obs. Hct}}$$
Ex Vol = the volume of blood to be removed and replaced, BV = blood volume (87 mL/kg in a term newborn), and Obs. Hct = the observed or measured hematocrit level.
5. Exchange is performed most easily via the umbilical vein using 10–15 mL aliquots after introducing a No. 5 Fr umbilical catheter far enough to obtain easy withdrawal of blood. This usually can be accomplished with a catheter insertion of less than 5–6 cm. Strict sterile technique is mandatory.
6. It is a difficult question whether to treat a child who is apparently asymptomatic with a high hematocrit level (greater than 70%). We favor treating because the risks of the procedure appear to be very slight, whereas the potential complications (microinfarcts of cerebral and other tissue) are ominous. However, if such complications already have occurred, the procedure will only minimize their extension. Recent evidence suggests these polycythemic children are at some risk of later developmental problems whether they are treated or not. The preliminary findings need much further confirmation.

7. The asymptomatic infant with a central hematocrit level between 65% and 70% also poses the question of whether to treat or not. There are no concurring data at present upon which to base a firm recommendation. Comprehensive follow-up studies are lacking, and what information has recently become available suggests a more limited role for partial exchange transfusions. Until more comprehensive studies are reported, this area will remain a very controversial one in pediatrics.

REFERENCES

1. Gatti R, Muster A, Cole R et al: Neonatal polycythemia with transient cyanosis and cardiorespiratory abnormalities. J Pediatr 69:1063, 1966.
2. Goldberg K, Wirth F, Hathaway W et al: Neonatal hyperviscosity II: effect of partial exchange transfusion. Pediatrics 69:419, 1982.
3. Gross G, Hathaway W, McGaughey H: Hyperviscosity in the neonate. J Pediatr 82:1004, 1973.

NEONATAL ANEMIA

GENERAL CONSIDERATIONS

1. Hemoglobin and hematocrit levels increase slowly from a mean of 14.5% and 45% at 28 weeks' gestation to a mean of 18% and 55% at term.
2. Hemoglobin composition is about 85% fetal at 28 weeks' gestation and about 65% fetal at term.
3. Diagnosis of a severe anemia in a neonate should trigger an investigation for other circulating cellular abnormalities, e.g., thrombocytopenia or neutropenia. All may occur together.

CAUSES AND DIAGNOSIS

Fetal Blood Loss (Extensive)

This results in anemia without jaundice in the first days of life.

1. Obstretic causes of blood loss such as abruptio placentae may result in fetal bleeding.
2. Fetal-to-maternal transfusions can be diagnosed by the Kleihauer-Betke test (smear of mother's blood to look for fetal cells in the maternal circulation). This is an important cause of unexplained anemia in the first hours of life.
3. Blood may be lost from a ruptured umbilical cord.
4. Repeated blood sampling in sick infants eventually results in anemia.

Fetal-Neonatal Blood Loss

1. Subdural or intraventricular hemorrhage often complicates a difficult or premature delivery. Diagnosis is made by a CT scan or sonogram or by aspiration of blood from the subdural space. A ruptured liver or spleen also may occur with traumatic delivery.
2. Hemorrhage into the lungs or peritoneal space occurs in sick infants, especially those with DIC.

Increased Erythrocyte Destruction

This produces anemia with rapidly developing indirect jaundice (see also Chapter 18). Causes include:

1. Isoimmunization (Rh, ABO, or minor blood group incompatibility).
2. Disseminated intravascular coagulation with intravascular losses. (See also section on The Bleeding Newborn, this chapter).
3. G6PD enzyme deficiency, which results in deformed erythrocytes.
4. Infection, which may produce erythrocyte destruction, although this is very unusual without other (usually many other) signs of congenital or acquired infection.
5. Red cell membrane disorders (e.g., congenital spherocytosis).
6. Angiopathic hemolytic anemias, which occur with cavernous hemangioma.

Deficiencies or Defective Production of Erythrocytes in the Marrow

1. Alpha-thalassemia produces severe hydrops, anemia, and often stillbirth. It is most common in Asian and Oriental children. Beta-chain abnormalities (beta-thalassemia, sickle-cell disease) do not normally produce anemia or other symptoms and signs of illness in the immediate newborn period.
2. Congenital erythrocytic aplasia occurs in an otherwise healthy infant with an abnormal decrease in erythroid elements in bone marrow. This is an important diagnosis to consider, as early steroid therapy may be beneficial. Diagnosis is confirmed by bone marrow examination. There is a 2:1 female predisposition to this disease.

GENERAL EVALUATION

1. Ongoing destruction of erythrocytes will rarely be reflected in a significantly low or rapidly falling hematocrit level without a

concomitant or preceding rise in serum bilirubin levels. The breakdown of each gram of hemoglobin results in 35 mg of bilirubin that must be metabolized by the liver.

2. There may be a delay in the hematocrit decline following sudden single-episode bleeding problems; therefore, serial hematocrit readings in the first 24 hr of life may be helpful. Anemia that is first detected at more than 48 hr of age is most likely hemolytic.
3. Clinical features of acute blood loss are hypotension, pallor, rapid pulse (more than 160 beats/min), gasping rapid respirations, and a low (less than 3–4 mm Hg) central venous pressure if measured via an umbilical vein or external jugular catheter inserted in the right atrium.
4. The reticulocyte count normally is elevated at birth (approximately 7%) and falls to 1–2% by the end of the first week. Severe hemolytic anemias are typically associated with persistently elevated reticulocyte counts.

TREATMENT

1. Anemia may be life-threatening at birth, as in Rh disease or severe fetal-to-maternal hemorrhage. It may require immediate transfusions with whole blood or type O negative packed red blood cells to raise the hematocrit level, treat the presumptive cardiac failure, and overcome poor oxygen tissue delivery.
2. Acute blood loss should be treated with a rapid infusion of 10–15 mL/kg of type O negative fresh whole blood. If this is not immediately available, restoration of intravascular volume can be accomplished with saline, lactated Ringer's solution, or 5% dextrose in saline. Treatment may have to be repeated, depending on clinical response (pulse rate, color), central venous pressure rise, and urine output.
3. A greater clinical problem in the hemolytic anemias seen in neonates is the management of associated jaundice and the selection of an appropriate maximum level of serum bilirubin for the performance of an exchange transfusion as the ultimate method of lowering serum levels (see Chapter 18).
4. Packed cell transfusions may be required after several weeks of life for infants with hemolytic disease, whether or not they received an exchange transfusion during the first days of life. This is because ongoing slow hemolysis will not be clinically evident as the jaundice diminishes, and these infants may develop high output congestive heart failure as their hematocrit levels fall below 15–18%.

ADDITIONAL COMMENTS

Anemia in the newborn is often an emergency requiring rapid transfusion, and it frequently reflects other significant illness (e.g., congenital infection). Neonatal anemias are often genetic, and therefore every effort must be expended to determine the causes, even if the appropriate (and sometimes very complex) tests must be deferred until the child is older.

REFERENCES

1. Gilman P: Hemolysis in the newborn infant resulting from deficiencies of red blood cell enzymes: diagnosis and management. J Pediatr 84:625, 1974.
2. Oski F, Naiman J: Anemia in the Neonatal Period. *In* Hematologic Problems of the Newborn, 3rd ed. Philadelphia, Saunders, 1982.

THE BLEEDING NEWBORN

GENERAL CONSIDERATIONS

1. Bleeding, like anemia, can be a manifestation of many different disorders and should not be thought of as a single disease process.
2. Infants that appear healthy and have no antenatal history of risk for severe illness may bleed in the first days from previously undiagnosed inherited coagulation deficits (hemophilia), from failure to administer vitamin K at birth to promote hepatic production of coagulation factors with short half-lives, or from acquired platelet deficits. Sick infants with respiratory distress or sepsis who develop bleeding most often suffer from disseminated intravascular coagulation (DIC).
3. There is an incomplete understanding of the role of circulating anticoagulants in bleeding diseases in neonates. Some premature newborns with apparently normal coagulation studies will bleed fatally (pulmonary or CNS hemorrhage).

SPECIFIC DISORDERS

Inherited Defects. Hemophilia (Factor VIII deficiency) and Factor V deficiency are uncommon causes of bleeding. Infants with these problems can present with intracranial or gastrointestinal hemorrhage or severe bleeding following circumcision. Umbilical cord bleeding is typical of severe congenital defects. Diagnosis is made by measuring prothrombin time, (PT) partial thromboplastin time (PTT), fibrinogen concentration, and (depending on those results) specific coagulation factor levels.

Vitamin K Deficiency. Generalized hemorrhage can occur on the second or third day of life owing to low levels of vitamin K, a coenzyme vital for the manufacture of Factors II, VII, IX, and X. Marked depression of Factor II (prothrombin) on the second day appears to be critical in triggering clinical bleeding. Infants of mothers receiving phenobarbital, or phenobarbital and phenytoin, are at risk of bleeding on the first day of life because of vitamin K deficiency made especially severe by the anticonvulsant medication.

Isolated Platelet Disorders. Thrombocytopenia may occur as part of DIC, usually in sick children, but it often appears as an isolated defect. The most common clinical presentation is with the appearance of petechiae, but fatal intracranial hemorrhages also may occur.

Classification

1. Immunoinduced thrombocytopenia is secondary to maternal illness, especially systemic lupus erythematosus (SLE) or idiopathic thrombocytopenic purpura (ITP), which depresses maternal and fetal platelet counts by producing IgG antiplatelet antibodies.
2. It is also secondary to isoimmunization by platelet antibodies manufactured by the mother against fetal thrombocytes. These antibodies do not affect maternal platelets. Treatment, if indicated, is to harvest maternal platelets and transfuse them into the newborn. The condition may recur in later pregnancies. There is some question whether fetuses from subsequent pregnancies, if already thrombocytopenic, should be delivered by cesarean section to try to prevent head trauma and intracranial bleeding. Scalp sampling of fetal platelet counts does not always correlate with immediate neonatal platelet counts.
3. Maternal drugs, probably including thiazides, may cross the placenta and induce fetal-neonatal thrombocytopenia.
4. Inherited thrombocytopenia is sex-linked or autosomal.
5. Thrombocytopenia is associated with skeletal or renal anomalies (Fanconi's syndrome) and with internal or external hemangiomas that produce platelet trapping.
6. It may occur as part of organic acidemias in newborns.
7. Qualitative platelet disorders are a rare cause of neonatal bleeding, reported to occur in infants of mothers ingesting aspirin.
8. Isolated thrombocytopenia may occur secondary to necrotizing enterocolitis.

Treatment is to infuse platelets. The level of thrombocytopenia at which treatment should be instituted is usually stated to be

20,000/mm^3 even if there is no overt bleeding, and <50,000/mm^3 if there is any evidence of bleeding. In cases of immune thrombocytopenia exchange transfusions may be necessary to help control the problem, but the procedure has considerable risks of its own, including initially exacerbating the thrombocytopenia. *Very* fresh blood must be used to have any positive effect on the post-transfusion platelet count.

DISSEMINATED INTRAVASCULAR COAGULATION (DIC)

DIC is a generalized defect of coagulation that occurs in association with congenital or acquired infections, both viral and bacterial; obstetric complications; and severe asphyxia and hypoxia. As in adults with this condition, there will be evidence of intravascular erythrocyte destruction and prolongation of both PT and PTT reflected in depressed levels of coagulation factors, thrombocytopenia, and hypofibrinogenemia (sometimes less than 20 mg/dL). These abnormalities in coagulation studies may exist without clinical bleeding or may be associated with severe (even fatal) pulmonary, intracranial, or gastrointestinal bleeding. Table 16–1 provides typical normal values for commonly used coagulation studies for term and preterm infants.

Treatment is controversial. Besides treating the underlying causes, we recommend specific replacement therapy. Any platelet count in a newborn of <20,000/mm^3 should be treated with platelet-rich plasma; a platelet unit of <50,000 in a newborn with overt bleeding should also be treated. One unit of platelet-rich plasma may have a volume of 25–50 mL. This may pose problems of fluid overload if given to premature infants, but the platelets have a short half-life and must be given quickly. Additional or supplemental treatment will depend on the particular coagulation abnormalities encountered.

Fresh frozen plasma (10 mL/kg) will often help correct other coagulation factor deficiencies. Cryoprecipitate will help to cor-

Table 16–1. NORMAL NEWBORN VALUES*

	PRETERM INFANT	TERM INFANT
Prothrombin time	up to 22 sec	up to 18 sec
Partial thromboplastin time	up to 70 sec	up to 50 sec
Fibrinogen	150–300 mg/dL	150–300 mg/dL
Platelet count	>100,000/mm^3	>100,000/mm^3

*Normal values will vary between laboratories. We advise consulting the individual laboratory for interpretation of results and for any modifications in blood sampling or use of reagents because of the expected higher hematocrit levels in newborns.

rect severe hypofibrinogenemia. Platelet-rich plasma also contains significant levels of fibrinogen and Factor VIII.

Heparin has been recommended but never rigorously tested as a means of interfering with the vicious cycle of factor activation and consumption. Another therapy advocated for DIC is exchange transfusion, which offers the theoretical advantages of administering opsonizing antibodies and neutrophils as well as eliminating circulating toxins, but again caution must be exercised because of the high risk of the procedure in sick neonates. A recent controlled study (see Gross, Filston, and Anderson) indicated no special advantage in the use of exchange transfusion to treat DIC.

REFERENCES

1. Glader B, Buchanan G: Care of the critically ill child: the bleeding neonate. Pediatrics 58:548, 1976.
2. Gross S, Filston H, Anderson J: Controlled study of treatment for DIC. J Pediatr 100:445, 1982.
3. Scott J, Cruickshank D, Kockenov N et al: Fetal platelet counts in the obstetric management of immunologic thrombocytopenic purpura. Am J Obstet Gynecol 136:495, 1980.

17

GENITOURINARY DISORDERS

ACUTE RENAL FAILURE

GENERAL CONSIDERATIONS

In the absence of congenital renal abnormalities, oliguria or anuria in the newborn is almost always secondary to anoxia or cardiopulmonary disorders resulting in poor renal perfusion. A transient decrease in renal function is a common problem in critically ill infants, as approximately 25% of all infants admitted to a NICU will have some degree of acute renal failure. In the absence of severe congenital malformations (renal dysplasia and agenesis) of the kidney, most infants will have complete recovery of renal function as the primary disease resolves.

PRESENTATION

History. There is often a history of perinatal asphyxia that suggests acute tubular necrosis.

Concurrent Disease. Infants with severe hyaline membrane disease, persistent fetal circulation, or hypoxia secondary to pulmonary disease will most often have a diminished urine output over the first few days of life. Extremely LBW babies will have immature renal function with decreased glomerular filtration. Infants treated with indomethacin for closure of a patent ductus arteriosus will often become oliguric, with elevation of serum creatinine.

Evidence of Hypovolemia. This may not be accompanied by a decrease in mean blood pressure. Hypovolemic infants will often appear pale and waxy, with decreased peripheral perfusion and metabolic acidosis. Infants with severe respiratory distress syndrome or severe hypoxia will have a decrease in renal perfusion. Other prerenal causes might be inordinate blood loss, asphyxia at delivery, or congestive heart failure. Infants are not considered to be in renal failure unless the urine output falls below 1 mL/kg/hr, although flow rates below this level are occasionally normal. If anuria has been present since birth, then agenesis should always be suspected.

DIAGNOSIS

Blood Urea Nitrogen (BUN). Preterm >20 mg/dL; full term >15 mg/dL or an increase of 5 mg/dL/day. In infants in a catabolic state this increase may be greater.

Creatinine. Preterm infants <1000 g normal up to 1.5 mg/dL; full term infants <1.0 mg/dL. A rise of 0.2–0.5 mg/dL/day is suspicious for pending renal failure.

Serum Potassium. Greater than 7 mEq/L. Other electrolyte changes include an elevation of serum PO_4^- and Mg^{++} and a decrease in Ca^{++}. These changes are usually not marked.

Acute Tubular Necrosis

1. Urine sodium elevated.
2. Urine/plasma ratio of creatinine decreased.
3. Urine/plasma ratio of osmolality decreased (<1.0).

Prerenal Failure. To rule out, first establish an adequate blood volume and electrolyte composition, then deliver an IV fluid challenge of D10W in 0.25% saline at 20 mL/kg over 2 hr. If there is no urine, then try IV furosemide 1–2 mg/kg. The urine flow should increase within 2 hrs if there is prerenal failure.

Platelet Count

Obstructive Uropathy. Rule out by retrograde studies (see section on Congenital Malformations of the Genitourinary Tract, this chapter).

THERAPY

1. Establishment of urine flow may not alter the course of acute tubular necrosis, but it will assist general treatment (fluids and electrolytes) if oliguria is on a prerenal basis. Mannitol infusion has not proved helpful in critically ill neonates.
2. Fluid and electrolyte replacement: fluid intake should be restricted to insensible water loss plus what little urine volume is produced.
3. Hyperkalemia:
   a. Mild (≥6.5 mEq/L): consider enema of exchange resin (Kayexalate).
   b. Moderate (≥7.0 mEq/L) (peaked T waves): administer insulin 1 U/3g dextrose at 0.5 g/kg.
   c. Severe (≥7.5 mEq/L): calcium gluconate for ECG changes; peritoneal dialysis if pulmonary edema and congestive heart failure develop.

ADDITIONAL COMMENTS

Inappropriate ADH, secondary to asphyxia, may complicate the diagnosis and treatment of acute tubular necrosis.

REFERENCES

1. Anand SK, Northway JD, Crussi FG: Acute renal failure in newborn infants. J Pediatr 92:985, 1978.
2. Arant BS: Developmental patterns of renal functional maturation compared in the human neonate. J Pediatr 92:705, 1978.
3. Mathew OP, Jones AS, James E et al: Neonatal renal failure: usefulness of diagnostic indices. Pediatrics 65:57, 1980.
4. Norman ME, Asadi FK: A prospective study of acute renal failure in the newborn infant. Pediatrics 63:475, 1979.
5. Stonestreet BS, Oh W: Plasma creatinine levels in low-birth-weight infants during the first three months of life. Pediatrics 61:788, 1978.

CONGENITAL MALFORMATIONS OF THE UROGENITAL TRACT

GENERAL CONSIDERATIONS

1. Embyrologic development:
    a. The kidney begins development from the metanephros and mesonephros in the fifth week.
    b. The ureteric bud then initiates development of the secretory portion (failure results in renal agenesis or multicystic dysplasia).
    c. The wolffian ducts:
        i. Carry the ureter towards the bladder.
        ii. Form the internal male genital structures.
        iii. Become resorbed in the female.
    d. The bladder forms at 6 weeks of gestation.
    e. The urorectal septum divides the cloaca at 7 weeks.
    f. The urethra is completed at the end of the first trimester.
    g. Nephrons continue to form to 36 weeks.
    h. Urine formation begins at about 13 weeks (failure results in oligohydramnios).
2. Most congenital malformations of the urogenital tract are not easily treatable, since permanent damage has occurred.
3. Most malformations do not require urgent treatment.
4. Physical examination should determine whether kidneys are absent, displaced, or enlarged.
5. Gonadal dysfunction may accompany urologic malformations.

CYSTS OF KIDNEYS

General Considerations

1. An enlarged unilateral kidney detected as a flank mass on physical examination of the newborn is most likely a cystic lesion.
2. There are a large variety of cystic lesions:
   a. Multicystic disease is most common. It is unilateral and usually affects males.
   b. Adult-type polycystic disease rarely presents in the newborn infant (autosomal dominant).
   c. Infantile polycystic disease (autosomal recessive).
   d. Solitary cysts, multiloculated cysts.

Presentation

1. The kidney is palpably enlarged except when there is a solitary cyst with an irregular, nodular surface.
2. The infant generally appears normal.
3. Multicystic disease more often involves the left kidney than the right, and the fluid-filled cysts will transilluminate.

Diagnosis

Intravenous pyelogram (IVP): no excretion, hyperplasia in contralateral kidney. Abdominal sonography will demonstrate cystic structure. Observe for anomalies in the contralateral kidney (30%).

Treatment

Multicystic. None. Observe during neonatal period. The need for nephrectomy is controversial; in any event, it should be delayed for several months.

Polycystic. None.

Multiloculated. Later resection of large cysts.

OBSTRUCTIVE UROPATHIES: HYDRONEPHROSIS

General Considerations

Hydronephrosis is a dilatation of the collecting systems, calyces, or pelvis with the retention of excess urine in the kidney. It is usually a result of obstruction at the ureteropelvic junction, although 10–15% of cases may involve a functional obstruction.

Hydroureters are usually present when there is lower urinary tract obstruction at the urethral valves.

Ureteropelvic Obstruction

Cause. The uretero-pelvic junction is the most common site of obstruction owing to intrinsic stenosis and (less commonly) an extrinsic obstruction such as an aberrant renal artery.

Presentation. A flank mass is a major sign. There may be subtle signs similar to sepsis with poor feeding and fever due to a urinary tract infection.

Diagnosis

1. Urine: normal or increased white blood cells and increased protein. Hematuria is rare.
2. IVP with follow-up films at 4, 8, and 24 hr to detect delayed excretion.
3. Retrograde pyelogram and voiding cystogram to determine the site of obstruction.
4. Abdominal ultrasonography.
5. Renal scan—delayed visualization.

Treatment

1. Surgical repair of ureteropelvic junction stricture, preferably by pyeloplasty if unilateral. Decompression by cutaneous pyelostomy or nephrostomy is sometimes necessary.
2. Antibiotics depend on culture results. Duration is long term.

Prognosis. Depends on the extent of damage at time of diagnosis and treatment. Bilateral hydronephrosis is associated with poor recovery of renal function when diagnosed during the first few days of life.

Ureterovesical Obstruction

1. Diagnosis of ureterovesical obstruction is usually not made in the neonatal period.
2. It may be associated with a ureterocele (usually in females).
3. Timing of surgical correction is determined by the extent of calyceal dilatation.
4. Observe for development of a urinary tract infection. Treat with low-dose antibiotics.

Lower Urinary Tract Obstruction

1. Bladder neck obstruction may present with minimal signs in the newborn. However, early diagnosis is extremely important.

2. It is more common in male infants.
3. The valves of redundant bladder outlet mucosa are the usual cause, although there may be intrinsic stenosis of the urethral orifice.
4. Diagnosis:
   a. Clinical: flank masses and palpable bladder. Poor stream in males with difficult and hesitant voiding.
   b. Cystoscopy: cystourethrogram and retrograde pyelogram.
5. Treatment:
   a. Early surgical correction of urethral obstructions.
   b. Upper urinary tract abnormalities include tortuous ureter and hydronephrosis, which require close observation and antibiotic treatment.

Vesicoureteral Reflux (VUR)

1. This congenital abnormality does not often present in the neonatal period.
2. It is probably a ureteral bud abnormality that is genetically determined. Siblings of affected infants have a 25% increased risk of developing VUR.
3. Half of all infants with urinary tract infections will have reflux.
4. It may be associated with other anomalies, such as renal dysplasia, posterior urethral valves, or imperforate anus.
5. Diagnosis: cystography.
6. Treatment: ampicillin and gentamicin when accompanied by signs of sepsis. Use long term low dose antibiotics as prophylaxis. Corrective surgery is indicated if an obstructive lesion is demonstrated.

RENAL AGENESIS—POTTER'S SYNDROME

General

Incidence is 1/4000 live births. The victims are almost always male. A large number are stillborn. The major associated anomaly is hypoplasia of the lungs. Other anomalies include gastrointestinal atresia, absence of internal genitalia, one umbilical artery, caudal anomalies, and amnion nodosum (see also Chapter 9).

Presentation

1. Potter's facies—abnormal facies with a wizened look, low-set ears, a small mandible, the nose flattened and turned down, and skin creases under eyes. Abnormal facies are probably secondary to oligohydramnios and in utero compression.
2. SGA status.

3. Immediate respiratory distress.
4. History of oligohydramnios.

Treatment

There is no treatment. Infants expire of respiratory failure in hours or days.

EXSTROPHY OF THE BLADDER

GENERAL CONSIDERATIONS

1. Rare: incidence is 1/50,000 live births.
2. It results from the failure of midline closure of the anterior abdominal wall, which affects the development of the bladder, urethra, and penis.
3. It is associated with genital abnormalities:
   a. Undescended testes.
   b. Absent vagina.
   c. Rectovaginal cloaca.
4. It occurs more often in males than in females.

PRESENTATION

1. Abdominal wall defect.
2. Ureteral orifices and urethra visible.
3. Pubic symphysis is widely separated.
4. Epispadias.
5. Inguinal hernias.

DIAGNOSIS

Diagnosis is clinical, by inspection.

THERAPY

1. Treatment is primarily surgical, with closure of the rami of the symphysis and plastic repair of the bladder in stages with ileostomies. There is some controversy over the timing of the procedures; however, closure of the symphysis is more feasible in the first few days of life.
2. Use saline pads to moisten mucosa prior to surgical repair.
3. Administer antibiotics.

18
JAUNDICE

GENERAL CONSIDERATIONS

Jaundice is the most common cause of concern in both term and preterm infants during the first week of life. The objective of treatment is to prevent kernicterus or CNS damage resulting from deposition of lipid-soluble unconjugated bilirubin. The objectives of management are to determine etiology, to assist in specific treatment, and to detect any underlying associated disease.

Several factors may be associated with an increased risk of kernicterus: LBW, prematurity, hypoxia, acidosis, and decreased albumin binding (e.g., as a result of drug interactions). It is important to understand the production, distribution, metabolism, and removal of bilirubin, since abnormalities at any stage of the physiologic process can increase serum bilirubin levels.

PATHOPHYSIOLOGY

Production

Seventy to 80% of bilirubin is derived from hemoglobin breakdown: 20–30% is derived from nonhemoglobin sources, such as rapid hemoglobin turnover in the marrow, or from the breakdown of myoglobin, cytochromes, catalase, and tryptophan pyrrolase. The average daily production of bilirubin in the infant (8–10 mg/kg/day) is approximately twice that in the adult. Red cell survival in the neonate is only 60–90 days. In addition, the newborn infant has a higher red cell volume and a larger proportion of nonhemoglobin substrate. One g of hemoglobin, when broken down, will produce 35 mg of bilirubin. The average full term infant will destroy red blood cells at the rate of about 1 g/day of hemoglobin or 1% of the circulating red blood cells.

Transport

1. Unconjugated bilirubin is released into the circulation by the reticuloendothelial cells and is bound to serum albumin.
2. One mole of albumin binds 2 moles of bilirubin. Additional but weaker binding sites exist. Tightly bound bilirubin is circulated to the liver, where the bilirubin is transferred across the cell membrane of the hepatocyte.
3. There is a wide range of binding; saturation may occur between 4 and 8 mg of bilirubin per g of albumin.

4. Factors affecting affinity are unclear and may vary with different degrees of oxygenation and among sick and well infants and premature and full term infants.
5. The distribution of bilirubin is determined by competing binding sites. The clinical appearance of jaundice is due to the binding of bilirubin to elements in the skin, presumably collagen. Adipose tissue competes with albumin for bilirubin. A number of drugs and endogenous substances, such as sulfonamides and free fatty acids, may potentiate the transfer of bilirubin from serum to tissue. Premature infants with relatively little fat may have smaller bilirubin stores and higher serum concentrations than full-term infants.

Metabolism

1. The mechanism by which the liver cells selectively remove bilirubin from albumin is unknown.
2. Glucuronidation in the liver is illustrated in Table 18–1.

Table 18–1. GLUCURONIDATION

Conjugated bilirubin (albumin)
↓
Hepatocyte (receptor)
↓
Unconjugated bilirubin + uridine diphosphate (UDP) + glucose (G)
↓
Unconjugated bilirubin + UDPG
↓
Bilirubinglucuronide (conjugated) + UDP
↓
Bile → reabsorption
↓
Excretion

3. Y and Z proteins act as intracellular carriers of bilirubin in the liver. The Y protein has greater affinity for bilirubin than the Z protein. It is unknown whether physiologic hyperbilirubinemia results from decreased glucuronyl tranferase, Y and Z carrier protein concentrations, or both.
4. The rate-limiting step in bilirubin disposition in the first 2 days of life is the hepatic conjugation of bilirubin, which is about 5% of the adult capacity.

Excretion

1. Once the bilirubin is conjugated within the liver, it is excreted into the bile and thence into the small bowel.
2. Reabsorption of bilirubin through the enterohepatic circulation results from increased activity of deconjugation by beta-glu-

curonidase, absence of bacterial flora, and decreased intestinal motility. As a result, deconjugated bilirubin can be reabsorbed and contribute to jaundice.

ETIOLOGY

1. Increased production of bilirubin:
   a. Hemolysis.
      i. Isoimmune hemolytic disease (Rh or ABO incompatibility).
      ii. Minor blood groups (Kell, Duffy).
      iii. Inherited red blood cell metabolic disorders (G6PD or pyruvate kinase [P-K] deficiency).
      iv. Infections (congenital or acquired).
   b. Polycythemia.
   c. Sequestered blood (enclosed space hemorrhage or swallowed maternal blood).
   d. Increased hepatic heme catabolism (starvation, epinephrine).
2. Metabolic disturbances:
   a. Glucuronyl transferase deficiency (prematurity).
   b. Inadequate Y and Z protein function (prematurity).
   c. Breast milk—pregnanediol derivatives.
   d. Hypothyroidism.
   e. Crigler-Najjar syndrome.
   f. Maternal diabetes.
   g. Hypoglycemia.
   h. Galactosemia.
   i. Drugs—oxytocin.
   j. Lucey-Driscoll syndrome (familial).
3. Increased enterohepatic shunt:
   a. High intestinal obstruction.
   b. Delayed feeding.
   c. Pyloric stenosis.
4. Decreased excretion:
   a. Liver disease:
      i. Biliary atresia.
      ii. Infections (viral, protozoal, bacterial).
      iii. $Alpha_1$-antitrypsin deficiency.
      iv. Dubin-Johnson syndrome.
      v. Rotor's syndrome.
   b. Drugs.
   c. Hypoxia.
   d. Erythroblastosis.
   e. Choledochal cyst.

PRESENTATION

Physiologic Jaundice

There is a normal transient elevation in serum bilirubin during the first week of life owing to the causes listed under Pathophysiology, e.g., increased red cell destruction, decreased glucuronyl tranferase in the liver, decreased hepatic transport of bilirubin, and increased enterohepatic shunt. Physiologic jaundice may be prolonged in premature infants.

Definition. Jaundice with a serum bilirubin of less than 12 mg/dL. However, a wide range of normal values for full term and premature infants has been reported.

Hemolytic Disease

1. Isoimmune antibodies against fetal red blood cells result in hemolysis of fetal red cells and increased bilirubin production.
2. An Rh negative mother may be sensitized to an Rh positive fetus; similarly, a mother with blood type O may be sensitized to A or B antigens entering her circulation from the fetus.
3. Other incompatibilities between minor blood groups include Kell-Duffy, among others.
4. Inherited red blood cell metabolic disorders include G6PD deficiency. It occurs most commonly in males and among Sephardic Jews, Greeks, Iranians, Sardinians, Chinese, Malayans, Fililpinos, and Indonesians. Approximately 10% of American black males are affected. In the newborn, it is usually not severe; it is rarely a source of jaundice, and it is generally accompanied by minimal anemia. The onset of jaundice is usually delayed beyond the second or third day of life.
5. P-K deficiency is an unusual cause of jaundice. Other rare cases are associated with 2,3-diphosphoglycerate mutase deficiency or 6-phosphogluconic dehydrogenase deficiency.

Delayed or Protracted Jaundice

Physiologic jaundice is often prolonged through the second week of life in premature infants, especially those that have been critically ill. In other infants, jaundice persisting beyond the second week should raise the suspicion of nonphysiologic causes, including:

1. Hemolytic disease (previously undetected).
2. Hypothyroidism (check T_4 screening level).
3. Breast milk inhibitors of conjugation.
4. Crigler-Najjar syndrome.
5. Pyloric stenosis.

Obstructive or Mixed Jaundice

Elevation of direct-reacting (conjugated) bilirubin occurs with severe Rh disease (formerly known as inspissated bile syndrome), usually following moderately high levels of unconjugated bilirubin. After phototherapy, infants with this condition sometimes develop a bronze appearance. The direct fraction gradually subsides over several weeks.

Sepsis resulting from *Escherichia coli* may present rarely, with a high direct bilirubin level in the second week of life. The TORCH (toxoplasmosis, rubella, CMV, herpes simplex virus) group of infections can cause liver disease, as can coxsackievirus B infections. These congenital infections often cause hepatosplenomegaly, thombocytopenia, and intrauterine growth retardation (IUGR). Galactosemia may result in mixed jaundice after the first week of life owing to hemolysis and liver damage from ingested galactose.

DIAGNOSIS

History

Check the family history and previous siblings (see list of possible etiologies).

Clinical

Hepatosplenomegaly, anemia, edema, hydrops, vomiting, regurgitation, cephalhematoma, and petechiae may be associated with jaundice.

Laboratory

A serum bilirubin level exceeding 7 mg/dL on day 1, 9 mg/dL on day 2, or 11 mg/dL on day 3 or thereafter necessitates at the least the following tests:

1. Red blood cell smear (spherocytes).
2. Blood type, Rh, and Coombs' tests for mother and infant.
3. Hematocrit.

Additional tests include:

1. Platelet count (thrombocytopenia occurs in severe infections and Rh disease).
2. Reticulocyte count (> 6% indicates increased production).
3. Serum albumin (a rough guide to binding capacity).
4. Liver function studies—SGOT, alkaline phosphatase (mixed or obstructive jaundice).
5. T_4 (prolonged jaundice).
6. Culture or serologic screen for congenital viral infections.

7. Urine-reducing substances (galactosemia).
8. $Alpha_1$-antitrypsin.
9. Sweat chloride.
10. Red cell enzymes (G6PD, P-K).

Determination of free bilirubin (horseradish peroxidase method) is not sufficiently tested to provide management guidelines. Binding studies have not proved reliable in determining risk for kernicterus.

MANAGEMENT

Phototherapy

Photoisomerization of bilirubin through the skin is an acceptable (if not overused) method of treating jaundice. The object is to obviate the need for an exchange transfusion and decrease the risk for kernicterus. Since the criteria for exchange transfusion and the risk of kernicterus vary with gestational age, birth weight, and antecedant or existing hypoxia or acidosis, it is difficult to recommend a specific bilirubin concentration at which to begin phototherapy. Some rough guidelines follow.

Guidelines. There is a risk of kernicterus when:

1. Indirect bilirubin > 8 mg/dL in < 1000 g infants.
2. Indirect bilirubin>7 mg/dL in very LBW infants and those with isiommune hemolytic disease (first day) or enclosed hemorrhage (bruising).
3. Bilirubin > 13 mg/dL in a healthy infant with a threshold for exchange transfusion at 20 mg/dL.
4. For intermediate levels (7–13 mg/dL) initiation of phototherapy is dictated by birth weight, concurrent illness, and postnatal age.

Methods

1. Use white light.
2. Check the intensity or change bulbs regularly (425–475 nm is the proper wavelength range).
3. Cover the eyes.
4. Monitor the core temperature q 2–4 hr, depending on birth weight.
5. Calculate a 50% increase in insensible water loss.
6. Measure serum bilirubin levels q 12 hr.
7. Discontinue if there is high direct bilirubin.
8. Be alert to the underlying disease described earlier in this chapter.
9. Follow hematocrit readings to detect hemolysis.

Exchange Transfusion

The exact threshold for exchange transfusion will depend on other variables influencing the risk for kernicterus, including severity of illness, acidosis, age, birth weight, gestational age, and Apgar score.

Guidelines

1. A full term healthy infant (>2500 g) without hemolytic-induced jaundice is probably not at risk for kernicterus with bilirubin levels below 22–24 mg/dL.
2. A full term infant with respiratory distress or a history of hypoxia is at risk at 18 mg/dL.
3. Infants 1501–2500 g—healthy 18–19 mg/dL, ill 15–17 mg/dL.
4. Infants 1001–1500 g—healthy 13–15 mg/dL, ill 13 mg%.
5. Infants less than 1000 g—healthy 11–12 mg/dL, ill 9–11 mg/dL.

Methods

1. Use fresh whole blood crossmatched with that of the mother. If the infant is Rh sensitive, use Rh negative and ABO specific blood, e.g., type O Rh negative cells resuspended in AB plasma.
2. Use anticoagulated blood—acid citrate dextrose (ACD) or, preferably, citrate phosphate dextrose (CPD).
3. Calculate blood volume (87 mL/kg at term or 100 mL/kg for approximately 1000 g birth weight), and plan on a 2 volume exchange.
4. Clear thrombi from a blood vessel and insert a catheter using aseptic technique. If a venous catheter is used, maintain sterility so that the catheter can be repositioned during the procedure.
5. Place the catheter in the umbilical vein or umbilical artery. In an older full term infant, the umbilical vein is preferable.
6. Heat the blood by passing it through a heat exchanger.
7. Monitor ECG, respiration, temperature, and color.
8. Provide an external heat source.
9. Empty the stomach.
10. Use aliquots of 5–15 mL of blood, depending on infant's size and cardiovascular stability.
11. Measure venous pressure periodically.
12. The time of exchange transfusion should be approximately 2 hr.
13. Albumin (1 g/kg 1–2 hr prior to exchange transfusion) is optional in a full term infant with Rh disease who is otherwise well.
14. Check ECG strip for tachycardia or bradycardia.
15. Calcium gluconate (2 mL 5% q 100 mL) is optional. Rinse

catheter with 1 mL saline before and after calcium. Calcium may not be necessary if the ECG is monitored closely.

16. Remove the venous catheter after the procedure. Leave the arterial catheter in the vessel with a glucose infusion running.
17. Monitor vital signs q 1 hr over the next 12–24 hr.
18. Use the withdrawal as sample for hematocrit and bilirubin levels, which should be monitored immediately after the exchange, then at 1 hr, and then at 8–12 hr intervals.
19. Use Dextrostix or Chemstrip to test for reactive hypoglycemia.
20. Determine pH 1 hr after exchange. The metabolism of acid citrate or dextrose phosphate can result in alkalosis.

Complications

1. Embolism.
2. Arrhythmias.
3. Increased potassium and sodium; decreased ionized calcium and glucose.
4. Infection (sepsis, hepatitis, CMV).

REFERENCES

1. Hegyi T, Polin RA, Driscoll JM Jr: Conjugated hyperbilirubinemia in infants with erythroblastosis fetalis. Am J Gastroenterol 72:297, 1979.
2. Levine RL: Bilirubin: worked out years ago? Pediatrics 64:380, 1979.
3. Lucey JF: Bilirubin and brain damage—a real mess. Pediatrics 69:382, 1982.
4. Maisels MJ: Neonatal Jaundice. *In* Avery GB (ed): Neonatology, Pathophysiology, and Management of the Newborn, 2nd ed. Philadelphia, Lippincott, 1981.
5. McDonagh AF: Phototherapy: a new twist to bilirubin. J Pediatr 72:297, 1979.
6. Wood B, Culley P, Roginski C et al: Factors affecting neonatal jaundice. Arch Dis Child 54:111, 1979.

19

INFANT OF THE DIABETIC MOTHER

GENERAL CONSIDERATIONS

1. Guidelines to the management of many of the problems common to infants of diabetic or gestational diabetic mothers are discussed in more detail elsewhere in this book. This chapter is a concise guide to the problems these infants may encounter.
2. Because there are a large number of diabetic women of childbearing age, the clinical problems of IDMs are sufficiently common to be seen in any delivery service or nursery.
3. The strict control of maternal glucose levels, especially during the last trimester of pregnancy, may limit or ameliorate the risk of certain complications in the newborn, especially those associated with fetal macrosomia; but it has not yet been proved that such management can also reduce the high incidence of congenital malformations found in these infants. If strict maternal glucose control were useful in minimizing the risk of malformations, it would be necessary from the beginning of pregnancy.
4. Infants of diabetic fathers are not at risk for this constellation of problems.

PATHOPHYSIOLOGY

Much experimental evidence has now been accumulated to confirm that maternal (and hence fetal) hyperglycemia provokes fetal pancreatic beta-cell hyperplasia and fetal and neonatal hyperinsulinemia. This occurs because glucose crosses the placenta and insulin does not. The excessive fetal insulin secretion promotes excessive growth of certain organs, especially the heart, adrenals, liver, and adipose tissue. The circulating erythrocyte mass is also increased in the IDM. This functional hyperinsulinemia is also partly but probably not wholly responsible for neonatal hypoglycemia.

Severe long-standing maternal diabetes is associated with maternal vascular disease and uteroplacental insufficiency. This chronic problem of pregnancy is associated with undergrown infants—who may also be hypoglycemic, but for different reasons than the typical LGA IDM.

DIAGNOSIS

Diagnosis of an IDM is by maternal history, including an abnormal glucose tolerance test.

CLINICAL PRESENTATION

1. Typical somatic features:
   a. Overweight and (often) overlength for gestational age.
   b. Head circumference appropriate for gestational age.
   c. Hepatomegaly.
   d. Cardiomegaly.
   e. Excessive subcutaneous fat tissue.
2. Other features:
   a. Infants often alternate between lethargic and irritable states, not necessarily correlated with serum glucose levels.
   b. Infants may feed poorly during the first days of life.

COMMON PROBLEMS

1. Birth injuries occur commonly because of the large size of the infant (see Chapter 3).
2. Respiratory distress may occur in the first hours or days for several reasons:
   a. Diaphragmatic paresis or paralysis secondary to birth injury.
   b. Hyaline membrane disease.
   c. Cardiomyopathy. If congestive failure is present, propranolol may be the optimal treatment, as this entity produces a hypercontractile state and partial left ventricular outflow obstruction, a condition more likely to respond to beta$_2$-blocking agents than to ionotropic agents such as digoxin. Echocardiogram is necessary for diagnosis.
   d. Structural heart disease (VSD most common; see also list of congenital anomalies).
   e. Airway malformations.
3. Metabolic problems:
   a. Hypoglycemia ($\leq$30 mg/dL) may develop 1–2 hr after birth and may persist or recur during the first 48 hr, with or without symptoms (jitteriness, lethargy).
   b. Jaundice.
   c. Hypocalcemia.
   d. Polycythemia.
4. Significant congenital malformations occur in 5–10% of IDMs and include meningomyelocele, anencephaly, VSD, transposition of the great vessels, coarctation of the aorta, sacrococ-

cygeal agenesis, vertebral dysplasia, anal atresia, and renal dysgenesis.

5. Renal vein thrombosis may occur in these infants and can be diagnosed by palpation of a large flank mass or bilateral masses, and by the presence of oliguria, hematuria, and proteinuria.
6. A transient syndrome of "micro left colon" may occur, manifested by decreased stools and transient functional bowel obstruction, with distention and hence poor tolerance of feedings.

MANAGEMENT

The immediate problems are recognition of respiratory distress and institution of oxygen therapy and, if needed, assisted ventilation. If present, hyaline membrane disease follows at least as difficult and protracted a course in the IDM as in other susceptible infants.

The second immediate problem is monitoring of blood glucose levels. This should begin with blood glucose assessment by 1 hr of age. Assessment can be performed by single drop stick methods for heel blood. Monitoring can then be tailored to the individual situation (e.g., presence of other problems, symptoms of hypoglycemia), but glucose levels should be checked q 2–4 hr during the first 24 hr. Early (<3 hr) oral feedings may prevent hypoglycemia or treat asymptomatic hypoglycemia, assuming there is no concomitant respiratory distress. Some have advocated intramuscular glucagon to treat hypoglycemia in these infants, who have excessive glycogen stores, but glucagon may itself stimulate more insulin release, thereby eventually worsening the hypoglycemia.

Polycythemia should be diagnosed or excluded with a heel stick or venipuncture hematocrit test and treated; consider treatment if present (see Chapter 16).

ADDITIONAL COMMENTS

1. All metabolic abnormalities except jaundice diminish after 1–3 days. The infants become more alert and gradually improve their oral intake.
2. Improved obstetric management of diabetes in pregnancy should decrease the incidence of these complications.
3. The long term outlook is favorable for neurologic normality and ultimately normal body stature.

REFERENCES

1. Anon: Abnormal infants of diabetic mothers (editorial). Lancet, March 22, 1980, p. 633.
2. Cummons M, Norrish M: Follow-up of children of diabetic mothers. Arch Dis Child 55:259, 1980.
3. Mare S, Hirshfeld S, Riggs T et al: Echocardiographic abnormalities in infants of diabetic mothers. J Pediatr 95:1013, 1979.

20
SPECIAL INFORMATION

NEONATAL TRANSPORT

Neonatal transport allows clustering of critically ill newborns and young infants in centers that are adequately equipped and staffed around the clock. Pediatricians and obstetricians have made the most rational use of limited resources by regionalizing special care services for high-risk mothers and their infants, both unborn and newly born. Most regions of North America have at least informal (and in some cases highly structured and successful) consultation and transport services between hospitals that provide different levels of intensive or special care for newborns. We offer the following information to supplement that provided by local regional perinatal care teams.

THE TRANSPORT PROCESS

The decision to transport an infant depends upon a variety of factors including the availability of skilled nursing and respiratory therapists and equipment, x-ray and laboratory support, and the knowledge, time, and commitment of physicians. The following are diseases or conditions that might require consultation or transport.

1. Respiratory distress from any cause (e.g., meconium aspiration, neonatal pneumonia, hyaline membrane disease) if the hospital does not have the capability to monitor oxygen therapy and arterial blood gases or to give ventilatory assistance.
2. Intravenous fluid requirements that are likely to persist beyond 1 or 2 days.
3. Conditions requiring surgical intervention.
4. Infants less than 1500 g birth weight.
5. Suspected congenital heart disease.
6. Complications at birth, including depression and unresponsiveness to resuscitative efforts.
7. Infants of diabetic mothers.
8. Neonatal seizures.
9. Suspected infection (sepsis, meningitis).
10. Severe hemolytic disease.
11. Apnea.
12. Suspected shock.
13. Persistent acidosis of uncertain etiology.
14. Recurring hypoglycemia.
15. Infants not doing well for unknown reasons.

The following information should be made available to the consulting physician at the time of the consultation call once a decision to transport an infant has been reached.

1. Patient's name and age.
2. Parents' names.
3. Details of prenatal history, labor and delivery, and neonatal resuscitation.
4. Apgar scores.
5. Gestational age and birth weight.
6. Vital signs (temperature, heart rate, respiratory rate, blood pressure).
7. Oxygen requirements.
8. Laboratory work obtained (serum glucose, serum calcium, blood gas determinations).

The following should be ready to send with the transport team:

1. Cord blood specimen.
2. Mother's blood specimen (5–7 mL clotted).
3. Copy of mother's chart, including complete maternal history labor and delivery records.
4. Baby's chart with completed nursing documentation (e.g., urine, stools, vitamin K administration, prophylactic eye care).
5. Copies of radiographs already obtained.

Appropriate care of these problems by the referring staff will help reduce infant morbidity and mortality. The transport team should stabilize the infant as much as possible in the referring hospital before moving him. The stable baby has:

1. A patent airway and adequate ventilation.
2. Pink skin and lips.
3. A heart rate of 120–160 beats/min.
4. A rectal temperature of 37 C (98.6 F) and an axillary temperature of 36.5–37 C (97.7–98.6 F).
5. Metabolic problems corrected.
6. Special problems (life-threatening malformations) managed as well as possible.

Very LBW infants (<1500 g) are at increased risk for the development of retrolental fibroplasia and intraventricular hemorrhage. Therefore, take special care to avoid rapid fluctuations in arterial oxygen tension (maintain at 50–70 mm Hg) and systemic blood pressure (typical mean pressure is 30–35 mm Hg) in these infants.

MECHANICAL VENTILATION

GENERAL CONSIDERATIONS

1. Ventilators for use in patients weighing under 1000 g have been greatly improved over the past 15 years.
2. Most ventilators available for use in newborns are pneumati-

cally operated and have independent adjustments for controlling the duration of inspiration and expiration.

3. A perfect mechanical ventilator would be easy to set up and operate and would provide
   a. A constant flow of warm, humidified gas to allow effective spontaneous respiration.
   b. Intermittent mandatory ventilation within an easily adjustable ventilator rate.
   c. An accurate oxygen-air blender.
   d. An accurate positive end-expiratory pressure (PEEP) valve.
   e. A wide range of available cycling rates.
   f. A humidifier that does not overload the tubing with water particles.
   g. Very quiet operation.
   h. Rapid and accurate "feedback" information about pressure and rate measurements.

   No single machine meets all these standards; several come close.
4. Indications for mechanical ventilation (MV) for neonatal lung diseases are described in Chapter 9 in the section on Hyaline Membrane Disease.

PATTERNS OF VENTILATION

1. No single set of ventilator adjustments would be appropriate for all circumstances in which MV is applied.
2. There is no substitute for close observation of the infant's chest movement following attachment of the MV tubing to the intratracheal tube. There should be a perceptible (1–2 cm) rise in the chest cage with each breath; without this movement it is unlikely that MV is being used effectively.
3. Ventilator settings are matters of some controversy. For treatment of severe respiratory distress (HMD), many nurseries use one of two basic patterns:
   a. Rate: 20–30 breaths/min.
      Peak inspiratory pressure: 25–30 cm H_2O.
      Inspiratory-expiratory (I:E) ratio: 1:1 to 1:2.
      PEEP: 4–8 cm H_2O.
   b. Rate: 50–70 breaths/min.
      Peak inspiratory pressure $\leq$ 20 cm H_2O.
      I:E ratio: 1:1.
      PEEP: 4–8 cm H_2O.

   Each system has its adherents. Present evidence is too scanty to recommend unequivocally either pattern as likely to diminish the risk of lung or airway damage. Rather than adhere rigidly to one pattern, the physician should recognize that different dynamics and time constants (dependent on local compliance and airway resistance) prevail in different patients and at different times in the same patient. The physician must be flexible to achieve safely the goals of MV.

4. The goal of any pattern of MV is to normalize arterial blood gas tension (maintaining PaO_2 at 50–70 mm Hg, $PaCO_2 \leq 50$ mm Hg and pH at ≥ 7.3) while minimizing peak inspiratory pressure, mean airway pressure, inspired oxygen concentration, and the indirect effects of MV. (These side effects may include impaired venous return to the heart, impaired cardiac output, air leak complications, and the development of chronic lung disease or bronchopulmonary dysplasia.)
5. The key to adequate oxygenation in many parenchymal lung diseases is maintaining an adequate mean airway pressure (MAP). There are several ways of increasing the MAP to increase PaO_2:
   a. Increase the flow rate to produce a more rapid pressure upstroke. The chest fills with air more rapidly, approaching a "square wave" configuration when airway pressure is plotted against time.
   b. Increase the peak inspiratory pressure.
   c. Increase the PEEP.
   d. Increase the breathing rate.
   e. Prolong the I:E ratio.

   These maneuvers will have an uncertain effect on alveolar ventilation as reflected in $PaCO_2$. Each ventilator change should be accompanied by a check of blood gas tensions to document the anticipated event. An inappropriately high MAP can have deleterious effects on CO_2 and O_2 exchange.
6. A radically new mode of MV, high frequency oscillatory ventilation (HFOV), is currently under study as a potentially useful clinical tool. Tiny stroke volumes (less than the calculated dead space) are generated at rates of 5–20/sec imparting a vibrating appearance to the chest and often to the whole patient. The goal of this technique is to maintain satisfactory gas exchange with less distending airway pressure. It remains a strictly experimental technique at this time.

MONITORING

Monitors serve as an extension of close nursing observation. They constitute an "early warning system" to alert staff to important changes in vital signs and allow immediate response to potentially life-threatening changes in condition.

TYPES OF CONTINUOUS MONITORING

1. The most important monitoring in newborns is of the *cardiac rate,* done by recording the infant's ECG either from elec-

trodes taped to the chest at strategic locations or from tiny needles inserted into the intradermal layers of skin. Although extremely accurate for measuring the cardiac rate, these recordings are insufficiently accurate for more subtle ECG findings and should not be used for such purposes.

2. *Apnea* monitoring is most commonly accomplished by constant current impedance pneumography using the same electrodes as in cardiac monitoring. A low voltage constant current is passed through the chest cavity via the two electrodes. Chest movement modulates the current to obtain a component proportional to respiration. The absence of chest movement is detected; therefore obstructive apnea, in which chest movement occurs but no airflow is produced, will not be detected. However, airflow detection involves the use of intrusive equipment that itself may interfere with other aspects of infant care. We recommend never monitoring only for *apnea;* optimally, both cardiac and apnea monitors should be available.
3. *Blood pressure* should be monitored continuously if an arterial catheter is in place, both for knowledge of mean and systolic pressure values and as an alarm if the catheter is compromised. Such a system should allow for both continuous fluid infusion into the catheter and continuous pressure monitoring. A digital display of blood pressure and an oscilloscopic display of the arterial wave form are useful.
4. Continuous transcutaneous PaO_2 and $PaCO_2$ monitoring allows for noninvasive assessment of arterial blood gas tensions. Both techniques employ a miniaturized electrode attached to a small area of skin heated to 43–45 C (109.4–113.0 F), an electronic amplifier, and a recorder. Physicians have had more experience with transcutaneous O_2 monitoring ($P_{tc}O_2$), and such experience indicates that very good correlations exist between PaO_2 and $P_{tc}O_2$ as long as infants are not hypotensive, less than 12 hr old, or receiving vasodilator therapy. Arterial blood gas tensions should be obtained at the initiation of transcutaneous monitoring to provide an initial comparison with the transcutaneous value. Experience with $P_{tc}CO_2$ monitoring is not extensive, but initial impressions of its reliability are encouraging.

All four of the preceding types of monitoring require auditory alarms that can be set to signal both high and low values for heart rate, blood pressure, absence of respiration, $P_{tc}O_2$, and $P_{tc}CO_2$. Visual alarms alone are insufficient in a busy nursery.

INTERMITTENT MONITORING

Temperature

Infant temperature must be measured frequently. A variety of technical devices are now available to record rectal, axillary, and skin temperature. In addition, incubator air temperature must be recorded, as the infant's temperature will often fluctuate because of environmental changes.

Indirect Blood Pressure Measurement by Ultrasonography

An inflatable cuff with an ultrasonic transducer and a microphone is used. The transducer sends energy pulses above the audible range into the artery at the point of occlusion. As cuff pressure is reduced, these pulses are reflected back by the blood intermittently spurting through the artery—a sound detected with the microphone. The audible signal represents systolic blood pressure. Diastolic pressure is noted when the blood flow becomes smooth; it will be detected when the intermittent beeping of the signal is no longer heard.

Other Monitors

Other monitors include a temperature probe on the warming and humidifying device used for inspired gas, the air bubble alarm on constant intravascular infusion pumps, and pressure and gas flow alarms on mechanical ventilators. Failure of any of these devices can and has produced tragic consequences.

INDICATIONS

Any infant at risk for bradycardia or apnea needs to be monitored. This includes all premature infants of less than 34 weeks' gestation, all "sick" infants of any gestational age, and infants of any gestational age requiring supplemental oxygen therapy.

RISKS

The greatest risk of monitoring is that the potentially important message of the monitor will go unheeded. This may occur because the alarm signal was not placed in the "Ready" position, because the auditory signal did not sound or could not be heard, or because no trained person was close by to respond. Apnea monitors may fail to detect airflow stoppage if chest movement continues or if the infant moves about in the crib without breathing.

Minor risks include skin trauma from lead placement and skin irritation from the contact jelly used to obtain a secure electrical skin contact.

Withdrawal of monitors can pose a significant problem. An arbitrary protocol in use in our nursery suggests that monitors are no longer needed if the infant has sustained no apneic or bradycardic episodes requiring nursing intervention for 4 to 5 days. Many hospital beds are filled with otherwise healthy infants who are simply waiting out this time before discharge or movement into a less expensive environment. A single nurse's intervention to stimulate an infant may result in thousands of dollars of prolonged hospitalization costs.

SELECTED EMERGENCY PROCEDURES

ORAL INTUBATION

Equipment

1. See the list of equipment necessary in any delivery room, Table 3–1, p. 8.
2. Portex tubes (uniform internal diameter) may require a stylet for easy placement. Do not let the tip of the stylet extend beyond the end of the tube. See Table 3–4, p. 11, for the appropriate size tube.

Technique

1. Prepare the infant by suctioning secretions from the oropharynx and extending the neck with a diaper under the shoulders; draw the mandible forward.
2. Be sure the infant is lying straight.
3. Hold the laryngoscope in the left hand.
4. Move the tongue to the left-hand side of the mouth with the curved edge of the laryngoscope blade.
5. Identify the base of the tongue, then the epiglottis.
6. Gently lift the epiglottis up and away; directly beneath is the laryngeal opening.
7. Only after the physician identifies the laryngeal opening and sees the vocal cords should the endotracheal tube be advanced from the right-hand corner of the mouth (Fig. 20–1).
8. Avoid blocking the view of the larynx with the tube as the tube is advanced.
9. Avoid intubating the esophagus, which lies below the larynx and which will usually appear closed or collapsed during the intubation.
10. Slide the tip of the endotracheal tube 1–2 cm beyond the laryngeal opening.
11. Hold the tube firmly and do not let it slip up or down while withdrawing the laryngoscope blade.
12. Chest excursion and improved color and heart rate should all occur within seconds of effective ventilation via the endotracheal tube.

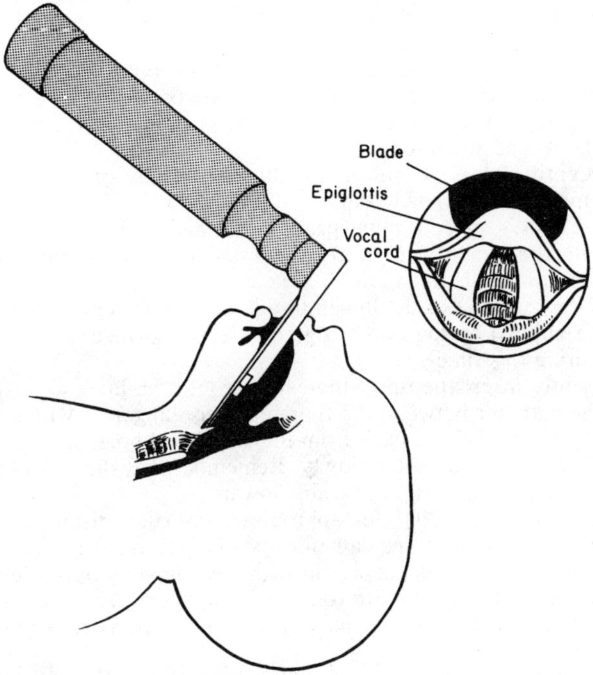

Figure 20–1. Schematic drawing of the technique of laryngoscopy for endotracheal intubation.

Precautions

1. Use a radiant heater and an electric heart rate monitoring device during the procedure.
2. Bradycardia is a signal to stop the intubation and resume ventilation by bag-and-mask technique.
3. Obtain a chest radiograph immediately to confirm tube tip position.
4. The metal laryngoscope blade is unyielding; apply it gently to all oral and pharyngeal structures.

UMBILICAL VESSEL CATHETERIZATION

Method of Insertion

1. Use all precautions for a sterile procedure, including sterilization of cord and periumbilical skin with iodine-containing solution.

2. Tie a loop of umbilical tape around the cord to control bleeding once the cord is cut.
3. Prepare the catheter and stopcock setup. Fill the catheter lumen with 0.9% saline containing 5 U heparin/mL fluid.
4. Cleanly cut the umbilical cord with a scalpel 1–2 cm above the top of the umbilical skin line.
5. Identify the thick-walled, usually constricted arteries and the single, more dilated vein.
6. GENTLY place a blunt probe or a pair of blunt iris forceps into the lumen of the artery. Do not try to insert the instrument more than 0.5 cm.
7. Allow the top of the lumen to dilate. Sometimes traction can be applied to the outer edge of the cut surface of the cord during this time.
8. Gently insert the tip of the catheter into the lumen, grasping the catheter between the thumb and forefinger or with a pair of forceps 1–2 cm back from the single end hole.
9. Advance the catheter slowly. Remember that the vessel runs initially caudad before turning inward.
10. Consult Table 20–1 for appropriate insertion distance. Two locations to place the catheter tip are (1) above the diaphragm and below the ductus arteriosus, approximately opposite vertebral bodies T7 to T10 (our preference) or (2) above the bifurcation and below the inferior mesenteric artery takeoff (L4–L5).
11. Secure the catheter with a plastic tape "bridge" and a suture around the catheter sewn to the skin of the umbilical stump.
12. Sometimes an umbilical venous catheter is inserted into the right atrium to monitor central venous pressure. The same technique is used. See Table 20–1 for the correct insertion distance.

Table 20–1. INSERTION DISTANCE FOR UMBILICAL CATHETERS (cm)*

SHOULDER (LATERAL END OF CLAVICLE) TO UMBILICUS	AORTIC CATHETER TO DIAPHRAGM	AORTIC CATHETER TO AORTIC BIFURCATION	VENOUS CATHETER TO RIGHT ATRIUM
9	11	5	6
10	12	5	6–7
11	13	6	7
12	14	7	8
13	15	8	8–9
14	16	9	9
15	17	10	10
16	18	10–11	11
17	20	11–12	11–12

* Data abstracted from Dunn PM: Localization of umbilical catheters by post mortem measurement. Arch Dis Child 41:69, 1966.

Precautions

1. Obtain anterior-posterior and lateral chest radiographs to confirm the proper position of the catheter.
2. The ideal catheter is easy to insert, totally nonthrombogenic, and radiopaque. Such a catheter apparently does not exist (yet).
3. Many complications may arise from the use of these catheters. Physicians inexperienced with such potential complications should not attempt to use this technique except in an emergency or for stabilization prior to transport.
4. Failure to pass the catheter almost always occurs because a "false tract" is created when the initial probing or the catheter tip itself breaks through the intima lining the lumen and is channeled into the surrounding tissues.
5. Failure of umbilical catheterization poses a dilemma for an infant in need of frequent arterial sampling. The physician's options then include attempting to enter the umbilical vessel via a subumbilical cutdown procedure, cannulating a peripheral (radial) artery, or maintaining transcutaneous monitoring with occasional correlating arterial punctures. Each choice has its own set of complications.
6. The insertion distances for catheters are only estimates. The tip may need to be repositioned following insertion.

LUMBAR PUNCTURE

Technique

1. Sterile preparation of the lower back is mandatory.
2. The puncture can be performed with the infant sitting up or lying on his side.
3. A small number 22 gauge, $1\frac{1}{2}''$ spinal needle should be used.
4. Advance the needle very slowly between the L4 and L5 spinous processes, toward the umbilicus. Remove the stylet once the needle tip is well through the skin.
5. As soon as fluid enters the needle, stop and allow spinal fluid to drain out.
6. Lumbar pressure measurements of the spinal fluid are of little use in neonates, and any attempt to take the measurement only serves to dislodge the needle.
7. The popping sound that occurs when the subarachanoid space is entered is usually not heard in neonates.

Precautions

1. A sick newborn is likely to require a lumbar puncture. However, the procedure poses significant risks to such an infant

because of the neck flexion and compression of the chest that occur while holding the infant to obtain a convexly curved back.

2. $P_{tc}O_2$ monitoring often shows a sharp fall in PO_2 during the procedure. Apneic and bradycardic spells are also very common.
3. When a lumbar puncture is needed to diagnose meningitis in a critically ill newborn with unstable vital signs, it may be advisable to delay the procedure and treat the infant presumptively. The lumbar puncture can then be performed later, when the infant is more stable. Duration of antibiotic therapy will then depend on results of a CSF examination (cell count) and concomitant blood culture results. Very few cases of neonatal meningitis occur without simultaneous bacteremia or septicemia.

PLACEMENT OF THORACOSTOMY TUBE FOR REDUCTION OF PNEUMOTHORAX

See Chapter 9.

SUBDURAL SPACE PUNCTURE

See Chapter 15 for indications.

Technique

1. Shave hair widely over the anterior fontanel.
2. Prepare a sterile field; prep with iodine-containing solution.
3. Use a short, beveled No. 22 gauge needle with a stylet.
4. Hold the needle perpendicular to the surface of the head and enter at the lateral corner of the anterior fontanel.
5. Advance the needle slowly, pointing the tip slightly medially.
6. The dura is rigid, even in newborns. A distinct "pop" or "give" will be felt when the needle tip penetrates the dura.
7. It is advisable to attach forceps to the needle just behind the tip prior to the final "pop" in order to prevent inappropriately deep insertion of the needle.
8. If fluid is present, it will run out through the needle when the trocar is removed.
9. Both sides should be tapped.
10. Collect the freely flowing fluid; do not attempt to aspirate it.
11. Remove the needle and seal the puncture site with collodion.
12. Serial daily punctures may be necessary.

ADDITIONAL COMMENTS

More commonly performed procedures (heel stick blood drawing and antecubital vein venipunctures) are better learned by direct observation.

DRUG DOSAGES

Tables 20–2, 20–3, 20–4, 20–5, and 20–6 are lists of the most commonly used emergency medications in newborn critical care. This listing of dosages does not imply that there is a thorough understanding of the pharmacokinetics of these substances in neonates. Some dosages are merely extrapolations from those used in adults, and greater knowledge of neonatal pharmacokinetics will likely change these recommendations. This listing represents data as of late 1981. It is not intended as a complete pharmacopeia but rather as a compilation of the most commonly used and important drugs for neonates. The listing of medications here should not be taken as proof that their efficacy in newborns has been finally established.

Table 20–2. DRUGS USED IN RESUSCITATION

DRUG	DOSAGE	ROUTE	COMMENTS
Na bicarbonate	2–3 mEq/kg	IV	Give as 0.5 mEq/mL, 1 mEq/min maximum infusion rate.
Epinephrine	0.1 mL/kg of 1:10,000 dilution (10 mcg/kg)	IV or, if no vascular access is present, via the endotracheal tube	
Atropine	0.01 mg/kg	IV, subcutaneous	For bradycardia induced by vagal stimulation.
Calcium*			
gluconate (10%)	1–2 mL/kg	IV	Slow infusion.
gluceptate (10%)	0.5–1.0 mL/kg	IV	Slow infusion. Watch for bradycardia.
chloride	0.15 mL/kg	IV	Watch for bradycardia.
Naloxone	0.01 mg/kg	IV, IM, may need to be repeated	To reverse narcotic-induced respiratory depression.
Glucose	2 mL/kg of 25% solution or 3–4 mL/kg of 10% solution, with frequent Dextrostix checks on blood glucose levels to insure adequacy of treatment.		

*See Chapter 13 for maintenance doses. No comparative studies in neonates have been done to recommend one of these forms of supplemental calcium in emergency situations.

Table 20–3. DRUGS TO COMBAT SHOCK

DRUG	DOSE	ROUTE	FREQUENCY	COMMENTS
Dopamine	5–20 mcg/kg/min	IV		Continuous infusion to correct hypotensive states once hypovolemia has been corrected.
Isoproterenol	0.1 mcg/kg/min	IV		Continuous infusion; tachycardia and further hypotension may occur.
Plasma-like substance	5% albumin in normal saline, 10–15 mL/kg	IV	prn	For correction of hypovolemia.

Other vasopressors may also have a role in treating hypotension.

Table 20–4. ANTISEIZURE MEDICATIONS

DRUG	DOSE	ROUTE	FREQUENCY	COMMENTS
Phenobarbital	10–20 mg/kg loading, then	IV		Therapeutic level of 20–30 mcg/mL.
	2–3 mg/kg	IV, oral	q 12 hr	
Phenytoin	10–15 mg/kg loading,	IV		Poorly absorbed orally.
	then 2–4 mg/kg	IV	q 12 hr	
Paraldehyde	0.3 mL/kg	Oral or rectal		Repeat as needed. Drug is excreted via the lungs, so caution is advised when it is used with coexisting lung disease.
Diazepam	0.1 mg/kg	IV		Antiseizure effect very short-lived; drug frequently causes respiratory depression.

Table 20–5. ANTIBIOTICS

DRUG	DOSE	ROUTE AND FREQUENCY (BASED ON AGE)	COMMENTS
Ampicillin	50–75 mg	IV, q 12 hr<1 week, q 6–8 hr>1 week	
Carbenicillin	100 mg/kg	q 8–12 hr<1 week, q 6–8 hr>1 week	
Chloramphenicol	25 mg/kg	q 24 hr for prematures, q 12–24 hr for infants >1 week	Follow serum levels; should be 10–20 mcg/mL.
Gentamicin	2.5 mg/kg	q 18 hr if <1000 g, q 12 hr if <1 week, q 8 hr if >1 week	Individualize dosage based on peak and trough blood levels—peak 8 mcg/mL, trough 2 mcg/mL.
Kanamycin	7.5 mg/kg	q 12 hr<1 week, q 8 hr>1 week	
Methicillin	25–50 mg/kg 50 mg/kg	q 12 hr<1 week q 8 hr>1 week	
Penicillin	50,000 U/kg	IV q 12 hr<1 week, IV q 8 hr>1 week	
For group B streptococcal infections, give a total of 300,000–400,000 U/kg/day in 100,000–150,000 U/kg doses q 8–12 hr if less than 1 week old or q 6–8 hr if more than 1 week old.			
Vancomycin	15 mg/kg	q 12 hr<1 week, q 8 hr>1 week	Slow IV infusion for methicillin-resistant staphylococci.
Moxalactam	50 mg/kg	q 12 hr<1 week, q 8 hr>1 week	Possibly of benefit against enteric gram-negative meningitis. Follow liver function studies.
Ticarcillin	75 mg/kg	q 8–12 hr<1 week, q 6–8 hr>1 week	Useful against Pseudomonas when used with an aminoglycoside.
Tobramycin	2 mg/kg	q 12 hr<1 week, q 8 hr>1 week	

Exact dosage and duration of therapy depend on the clinical state, the severity of the illness, underlying problems, and guesswork.

Table 20–6. OTHER DRUGS

DRUG	DOSE	ROUTE	FREQUENCY	COMMENTS
Indomethacin	0.2 mg/kg	Oral	q 8 hr × 2 or 3	IV form may be more effective for closure of the ductus arteriosus.
Dexamethasone	0.2 mg/kg	Oral, IV	q 8 hr	
Aminophylline	3–5 mg/kg loading, then	IV	Loading	Useful for combatting apnea.
	2 mg/kg	IV	q 8 hr	See Chapter 10.
Theophylline	5–6 mg/kg	Oral	Loading	See Chapter 10.
	1–2 mg/kg		q 6–12 hr	
Caffeine	10–15 mg/kg	Oral	Loading	See Chapter 10.
	5 mg/kg		q 12 hr, begin 12–24 hr after loading	
Morphine	0.1 mg/kg	IV	q 4–6 hr prn	
Pancuronium	0.05–0.1 mg/kg	IV	prn	Should not be used without concomitant sedation *and*, obviously, artificial ventilation.
Prednisone	0.5–1.0 mg/kg	IV	q 12 hr	
Digoxin Total digitalizing dose, oral	25–30 mcg/kg	Oral	Half dose to start, then	Preterm
	50 mcg/kg	Oral	¼ total dose q 6–8 hr × 2, then ⅛ total dose q 12 hr.	Term
Intravenous	20 mcg/kg	IV	Half dose, then ¼ total dose q 6–8 hr × 2,	Preterm
	30 mcg/kg	IV	then ⅛ total dose q 12 hr.	Term
Tolazoline	1–2 mg/kg to be infused over 10 min, then 1–2 mg/kg/hr	IV	Occasionally of use in persistent pulmonary hypertension.	
Furosemide	1–3 mg/kg	IV, oral	These diuretics will produce Na^+ and K^+ loss, and furosemide additionally produces Ca^{++} loss in the urine (increased risk for rickets when used chronically).	prn
Chlorothiazide	10–20 mg/kg	Oral		q 12 hr

INDEX

Note: Page numbers in *italics* indicate illustrations; (t) refers to tables.

NOTES

NOTES

NOTES

NOTES

NOTES

NOTES

NOTES

NOTES

NOTES

NOTES

NOTES

NOTES

NOTES

NOTES

NOTES

NOTES

NOTES

NOTES

NOTES

NOTES

NOTES

NOTES

NOTES

NOTES

NOTES

NOTES

NOTES

NOTES

NOTES

NOTES

NOTES

NOTES